Electrophysiocardiology

Wade H. Melvin. AAFP Diplomat

Jose L. Garcia, MD

Naomi F Melvin, PhD

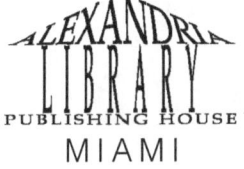

ALEXANDRIA LIBRARY
PUBLISHING HOUSE
MIAMI

FOREWORD

This book is basically aimed at medical and nursing students, residents and health technicians in general, although it may also be used for consultation by physicians and specialists. The basic fundamentals are presented in 7 chapters on electrocardiography through an eminently practical approach. A large variety of responses has been compiled, in addition to a careful selection of cardiovascular diseases that affect human beings. In particular, Chapter 7 deals with children's electrocardiograms, which are different than those for adults.

The contents of a technique that goes back to thee XVII is presented in a manner that is both summarized and didactic, based on the long academic career of the authors. The essential ideas are summarized systematically. Students must learn those ideas, in addition to learning how to interpret electrocardiogram results.

With the advance of technology, the equipment used in electrocardiography bring a large number of functions, including continuous patient monitoring, alert systems for abnormal conditions which are automatically detected by software, all the way to obtaining a diagnostic. However, in some systems, the automatic diagnostic does not match more precise clinical data because, in spite of all technological advances, the machine is still unable to fully replace the need for human interaction for the purpose of diagnosing, and that is due to the level of complexity of subject under analysis. For that reason, it will always be useful to be in command of basic knowledge that enables a person to support or reject an improper diagnostic given by a machine. In addition, manual reading of an electrocardiogram stills weighs significantly, in particular, in locations that are missing more precise equipment. Such ability is a life-saver.

It is necessary to bring electrocardiography to the level of the general practitioner, to resident physicians, to interns, to medical students, to nurses and, in sum, to all medical staff providing healthcare to patients in cases in which electrographic readings are necessary.

To summarize, the present text is being offered as a practical guide that integrates the knowledge of the electrical operation of the heart, all the way to the knowledge of how the several derivations are represented and the clinical interpretation of such derivations, while taking many anatomical and physiological aspects of the heart. The presentation of such knowledge is done in a manner that is both didactic and synthetic and, as such, this presentation brings a great deal of practical usefulness in learning to work with electrocardiograms..

El autors

TABLE OF CONTENTS

1   Electrophysiology

The heart is the main organ of the circulatory apparatus; schematically it is possible to be considered constituted by four cameras: two superior or right and left atrium, and two inferior or ventricles.

The right atrium receives the venous blood coming from various parts of the body through the superior and inferior venae cavae, and the left atrium receives the oxygenated blood that comes from the lungs through the pulmonary veins. From the atria the blood flows to the corresponding ventricles that are chambers constituted by a powerful muscle. The deoxygenated blood in the right ventricle is pumped through the pulmonary artery towards the lungs, where it is oxygenated, then returns to the left atrium and goes to the left ventricle to be pumped through the aorta to the systemic circulation, this oxygenated blood along with nutrients go to all the tissues in the body (fig. 1.1).

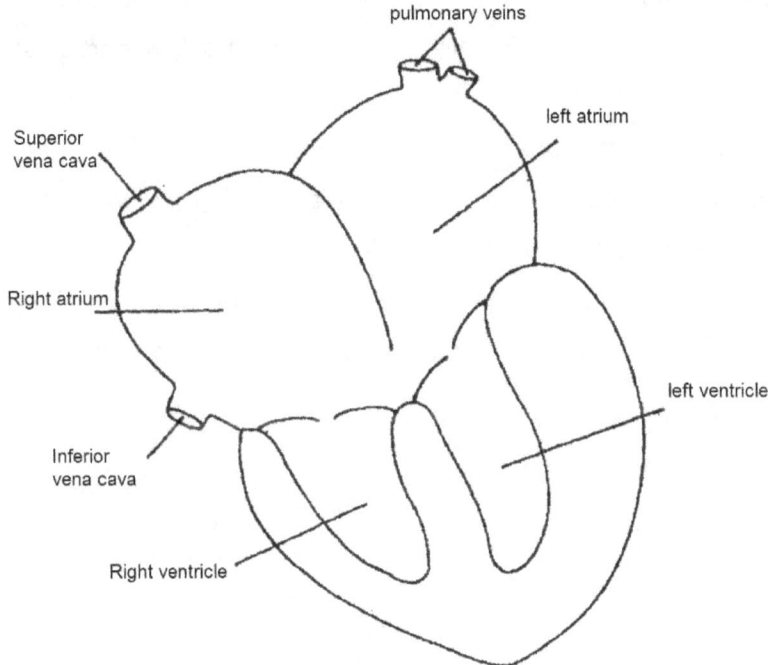

Fig 1.1 Schematic representation of the heart and its four chambers.

Heart wall

Three layers form the wall of the heart: the epicardium (external layer), the myocardium (middle layer), and endocardium, (internal layer).

The myocardium, which is cardiac muscle tissue is responsible for the pumping action of the heart.

Heart Conduction System

- Sinoatrial (SA) node or Keith-Flack node
- Internodale Fascicoli
- Atrioventricular (AV) node or node of Aschoff and Tawara
- Atrioventricular Bundle (Bundle of His)
- Right and Left branches of Bundle of His
- Purkinje Fibers and its branches

The sinoatrial node or Keith-Flack is located in the posterior and high portion of the wall of the right atrium, near the opening of the superior vena cava, this is the site where normally the electrical stimulus is generated and for that reason it is also known with the name of Pacemaker. The fascicoli internodale (anterior, medium and posterior) connect the sinoatrial node with the atrium ventricular node or Aschoff- Tawara, in the right and low part of the interatrial septum and then connect downwards with the bundle of His fiber, after a short passage, the bundle of His is divided in two main branches, right and left, that are distributed in the endocardial or internal surface of the corresponding ventricles and finish in the Purkinje fibers which them penetrate the endocardial surface of the ventricles.

It is important to know that the right branch of His does not subdivides, whereas the left one subdivides near its origin in two fascicles, one anterior and one posterior, which shorter and wider (fig 1.2)

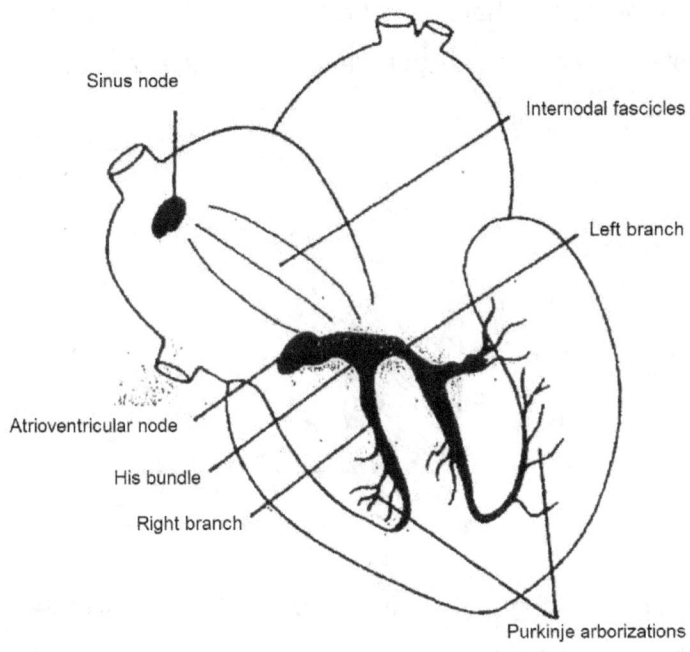

Fig 1.2 Schematic Representation of the system of conduction of the heart or specific myocardium

ELECTRIC ACTIVATION AND RECOVERY OF THE CELL

The genesis of the cellular electrical activity is determined by the presence of a series of substances like sodium, the potassium, the chlorine, the calcium, that are normally in ionic state, that is to say, they have small electrical charges and they are dissolved in the intracellular and extracellular space. If the cell is in a resting state, the positive electrical charges are arranged outside the membrane, whereas the negative electrical charges are in the interior; then, the electric field that surrounds this cell is positive in any explored point, since it depends on the electrical charges that are located outside the cellular membrane, and because they are all positive; potential difference does not exist, therefore, there is not electrical current. (fig. 1.3).

When the cell receives a stimulus in some point of its membrane, this becomes permeable to the ionic substances in that point, and the electrical charges spread through the membrane in the site in which it was stimulated, so that the negative charges go to the outside of the membrane and the positive ones penetrate in the cell. The electric field that surrounds the cell modifies and a potential difference appears, since in the site of the cell stimulation there is an

9

electronegative field, whereas in the portion of the cell that has not been stimulated, remains the electropositive field; this difference of potential causes the generation of an electrical current (fig. 1.4)

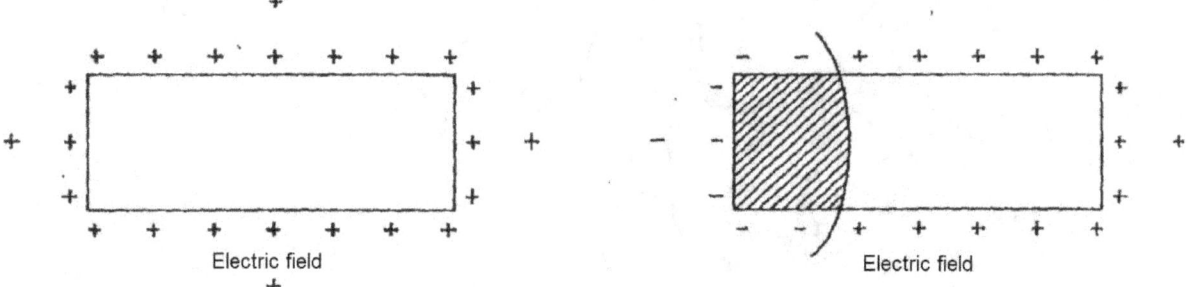

Fig 1.3 Cell polarized at rest. Difference of potential in the electric field that surrounds to cell does not exist

Fig 1.4 Cell in activation, the stimulated zone has created an electronegative field that establishes a difference of potential in the electric field that surrounds the cell and, therefore; an electrical current.

The described process does not remain static, is to say, from the point the cell was stimulated, advances towards the opposite side and totally activates the cell, that is, that the excitation wave is advancing through the cell, and it is possible to be compared to the progression of a wave that is leaving behind and electronegative filed, while at the front of his ridge it has an electropositive field.

The form of spreading the electric activation, makes that this phenomenon can be represented in vector form, where the magnitude or size of the vector shows the distance travelled by the activation wave; this is followed by a horizontal activation process, in this case; and the direction is recognized by the arrow of the vector, located to the left in the case represented, since the wave advances from left to right (fig. 1.5 a, b, c).

Immediately after the electric activation, there is a contraction or mechanical work, but for that cell to be stimulated, it needs to reorient its electric charges, so that all the positive charges are outside the membrane ie it must go through a process of recovery, that along with the activation process, can also be represented in a vector way by a vector in this case having equal magnitude and direction and sense that the vector of activation, but unlike the former, the electric charges are oriented upside down, since the electric field that is formed behind the wave of recovery is positive, while in the anterior portion or arrow of the vector there is an electronegative field (fig. 1.5 d, e, f).

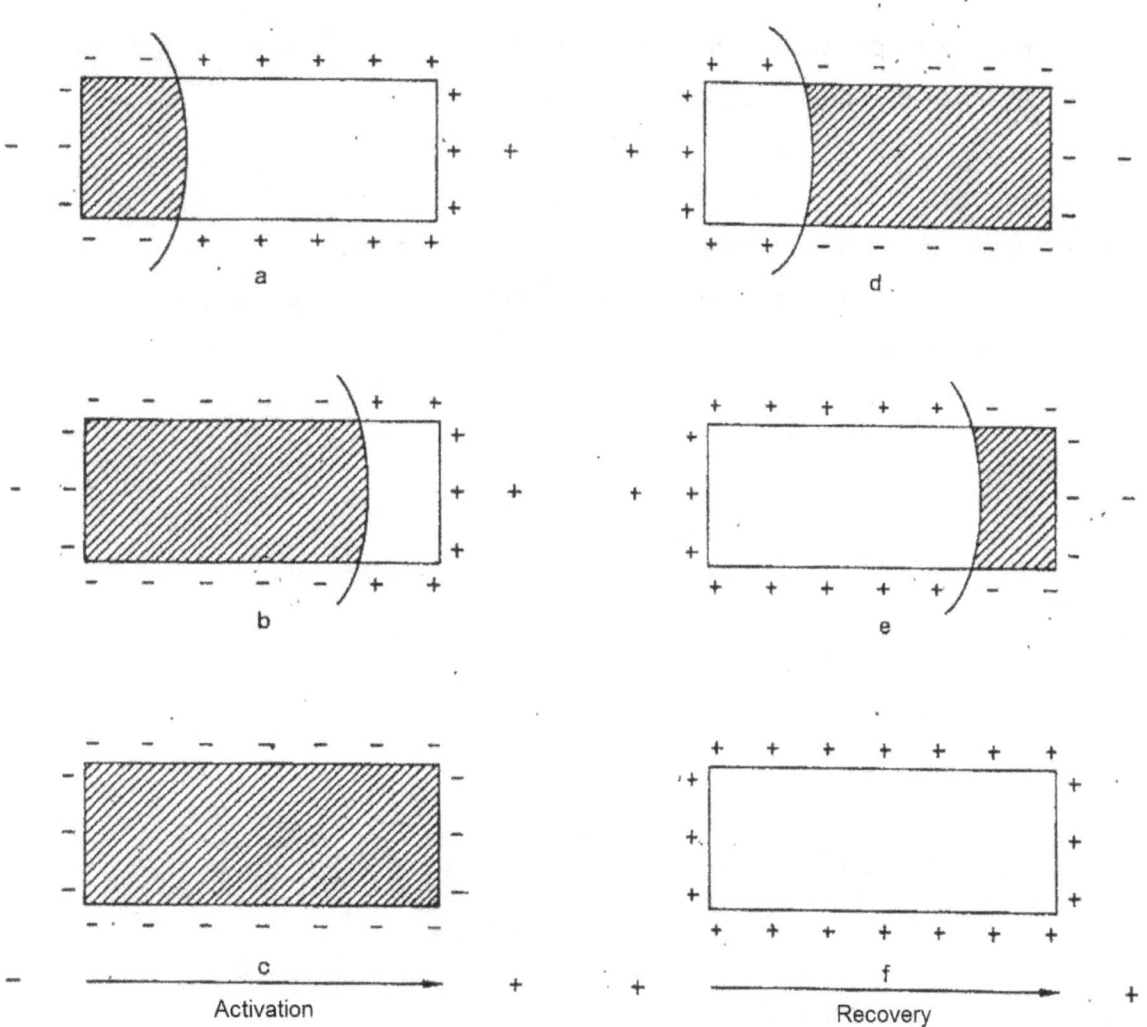

Fig 1.5 Activation and recovery process. For more simplicity only the electric charges have been represented on the outside of the membrane since they are ultimately the ones that influence the electric field.

The process of activation and electric recovery, are known as depolarization y repolarization respectively. This is due to the initially idea that electrical activation used to make disappeared all the dipoles formed around the membrane, and that in the recuperation such dipoles reappear again. Although the concept is wrong, the use has imposed this terminology.

GALVANOMETER

The galvanometer is an apparatus of electrical measurement used to determine the intensity of the current (fig. 1.6), schematically can be considered to be formed by two fundamental parts:

1. Box register, equipped with a pointer or rope, which deviates positive or negative according to the electric field where the electrodes are placed.

2. Two electrodes consisting of metal terminals which are those that explore directly the electric field; one of them is positive and the other negative. The more important is the positive and that is why is called exploring electrode; the negative electrode is named indifferent electrode.

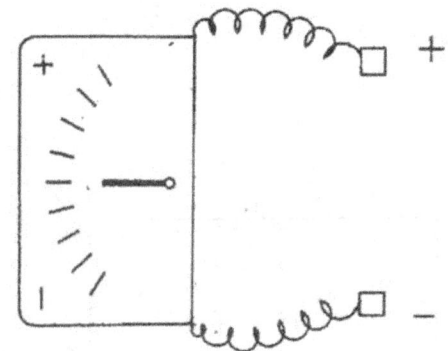

Fig 1.6 Schematic representation of a Galvanometer

Electrocardiograph is not more than a Galvanometer that has two features:

1. It is capable of recording minimal differences in potential

2. It has an enrolled grid paper where deflections or deviations from the needle or rope are recorded

To determine what type of deviation (positive o negative) is recorded in the draw, it is essential to know the electric polarity of the field where the positive or explorer electrode is. If this electrode is in a positive electric field, the deflection of the needle or rope will be positive, and vice versa.

Therefore there is a fundamental concept: every time that electric activation vectors have their arrow or anterior portion positive and a negative tail, the following will happens:

1. When the electrical activation wave approaches an explorer electrode, it will produce in the draw a positive wave, since the electrode is located in a positive electric field; the size of the wave is related to the intensity of the current, represented in this case by the magnitude of the vector (fig. 1.7a).

2. When the wave moves away from the explorer electrode, it will produced in the draw a negative deflection wave, since the explorer electrode is in a negative field (fig. 1:7 b)

When the route occurs in a perpendicular direction to the explorer electrode, it will produce in the draw an isodiphasic or equal to zero type deflections (fig. 1.7 c).

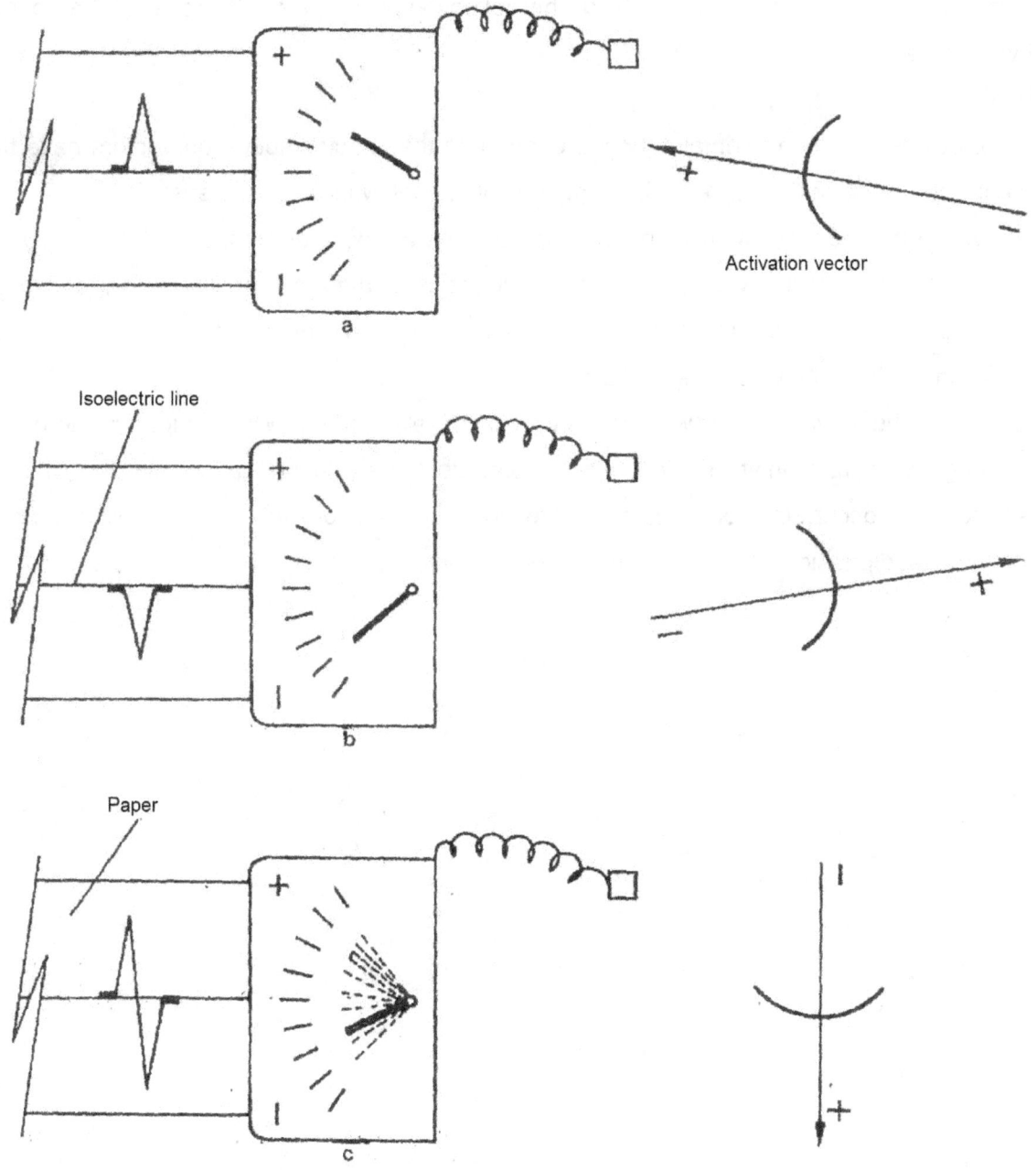

Fig 1.7 Representation of the different types of waves in the layout according to the route of the activation wave

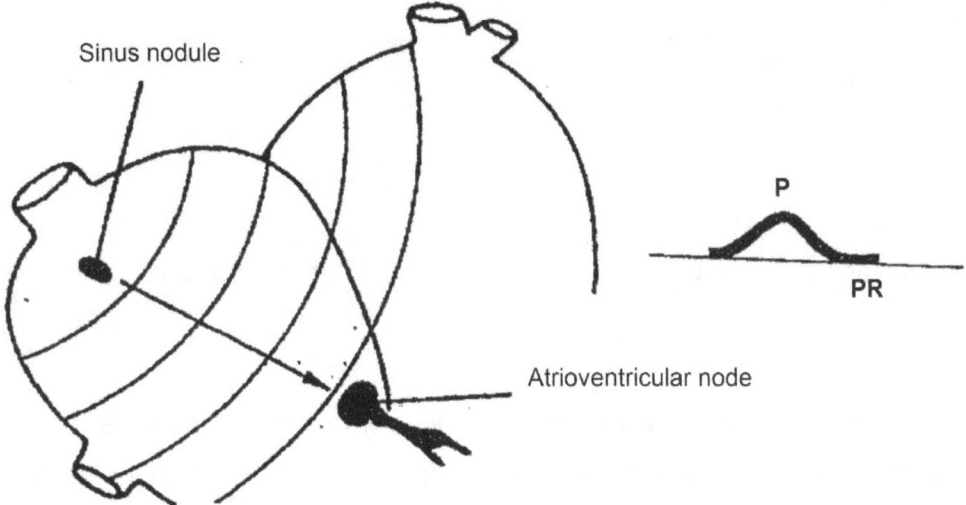

Fig. 1.8 Schematic Auricle activations by a vector oriented downward and to the left, which gives rises to the P wave in the electrocardiogram.

Once the ventricular auricle node is reached, the electric stimulus is retarded or delayed in traversing this node and the His bundle; in the electrocardiogram, that is shown by a thick trace that occupies the isoelectric line following the P wave and known as the PR segment (fig. 1.8) and that is the link between the auricular activation wave or P wave and the ventricular activation complex that follows.

After the electrical stimulus traverses the ventricular auricle node and the His bundle, it simultaneously penetrates through both branches and activates the ventricles, but, unlike toe auricular activation, which may be resumed in a single vector, the ventricular activation is represented schematically by three vectors, as will be explained next.

When the stimulus penetrates through the His bunch branch, the first ventricular portion that is activated is that of the middle of the ventricular septum, which is activated through the left His bunch branch and produces a first ventricular activation vector oriented left to right. That vector tends to be small (ventricular activation vector) (fig. 1.9)

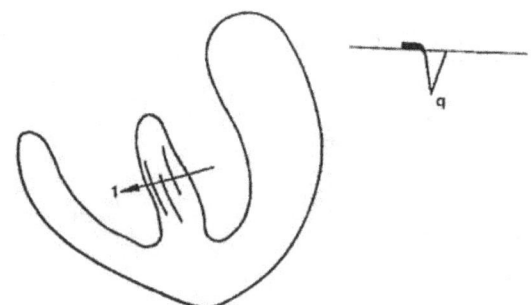

Fig 1.9. Septum activation. 1, the first ventricular activation vector that produces the Q wave in the ECG.

After the middle of the septum is activated, the stimulus or activation wave reaches the endocardic surface of both ventricles simultaneously and, at that moment, right ventricular activation vectors are produced, which move to the right; the left ventricular activation vectors move to the left; there also some vectors that move downwards. Now, this series of vectors that are generated simultaneously may be represented through a resultant vector (ventricular activation vector 2), which, by virtue of its larger magnitude and because left-oriented vectors, they tend to orient this vector down and left. This second vector that represents the resultant of the electric activation of both ventricles, median electric axis of the QRS complex. (fig. 1.10).

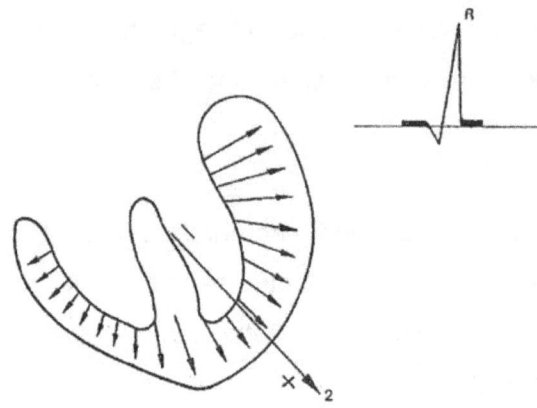

Fig. 1.10 Simultaneous activation of both ventricles, as represented by the resultant vector 2, which is responsible for the main QRS complex wave. The space orientation of this vector is the median electric axis of the QRS complex.

The last ventricular portions to be activated, due to the small amount of Purkinje arborizations they have, are those of the base portion of the septum and the posterior base of the left ventricles and a third, small vector is produced, which is oriented to the right and backwards (remaining vector or vector 3) (fig. 1.11).

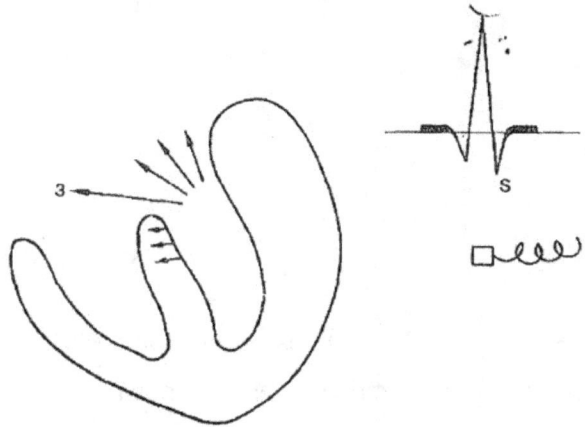

Fig. 1.11 Remnant vector or vector 3 of the ventricular activation, which is responsible for the S wave.

The three vectors, the septum vector or vector 1, the resultant vector or vector 2 and the remnant or vector 3, give rise of the QRS complex, which translates in the electrocardiogram in the electric activation of the ventricles; This electrical ventricular activation time is very fast,, generally. less than ten hundredths of a second (0.10 s)

While the QRS complex indicates the ventricle electrical activation, and has been represented schematically by its three waves, one needs to realize now that it is not always so, since you can have multiple variants in its form, which depends fundamentally on the angle or position from where it is picking up the electric activation. For that reason, is it important to know to recognize the waves, regardless of the morphology of the QRS complex. We have the following the following:

- The *R Wave.* These are all the positive waves of the QRS complex; if there are more one, the second wave will be named R.
- The *Q wave.* It is the first negative wave of the QR complex. It is followed by a positive wave.
- The *S wave.* It is the negative wave in the QRS complex that follows a positive wave.
- The *QS Wave.* This is the wave that results when only a negative wave is identified.
- (fig. 1.12)

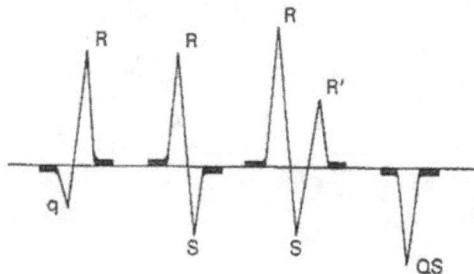

Fig 1.12 some variants of the QRS complex

After the electrical activation of the ventricles or QRS complexes is completed, the electrocardiogram a follows thick stroke hat occupies the isoelectric line and is known as the ST segment, which must be at the same level of its counterpart on the opposite side, the PR segment; is precisely at the moment when the heart is doing its mechanical work or contraction of the ventricles.

Immediately after the ST segment, comes the recovery wave or T wave; It is a slow-moving wave and therefore, it is a thick stoke, the same as the P wave; usually is a positive wave, although, as will be seen later, in some electrocardiogram leads It can be negative without implying any condition.

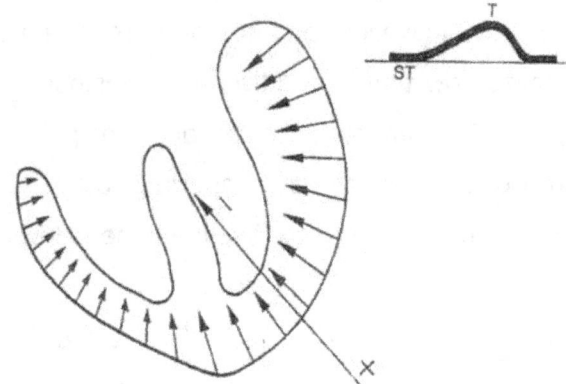

Fig. 1.13 Schematic representation of the recovery wave, or T wave.

2 Electrocardiography preliminary concepts

In the previous chapter the process of activation of the heart is analyzed and every aso This process is identified with the various waves of normal electrocardiogram Figure 2.1, but it is necessary to clarify that the P wave is the first wave of the route and is due to the activation Electric of the atria, the QRS complex is the result of electrical activation of the ventricles and need not be represented by three waves; the PR segment is the interval of time between the P wave QRS complex consisting of a thick line that occupies the isoelectric line and represents the time it takes the electrical stimulus to pass through the AV node and the bundle of His, the ST segment is a broad stroke that occupies the isoelectric line between the QRS complex (ventricular activation complex) recovery wave or wave T, and T wave is the T wave is the wave of ventricular recovery thick line and slow registration, whose positive or negative orientation, you must match the orientation of the QRS complex.

Paper for electrocardiogram

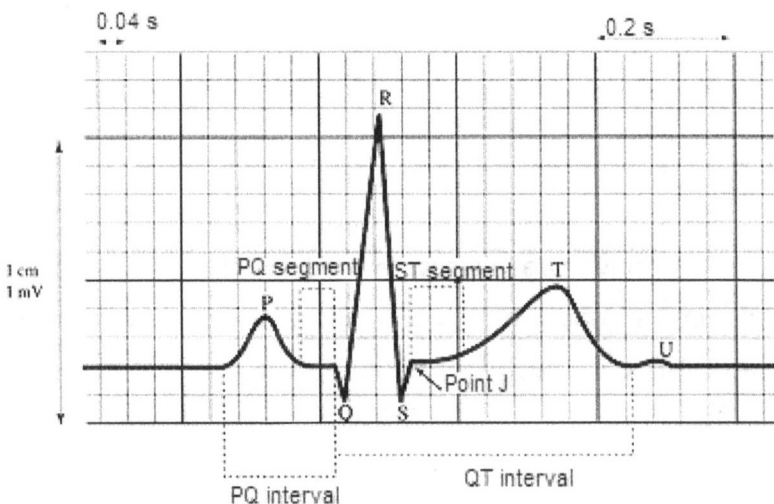

Fig 2.1 Different components or waves of a normal electrocardiogram

The paper on which is inscribed the electrocardiographic tracing is squared and graph; It is a series of vertical and horizontal lines. Each line to the next, the same in one direction than another is a millimeter away, and every 5 stroke is thick lines in order to facilitate reading; that is, that the paper consists of small cubes having a millimeter on each side and large squares of 5 mm per side.

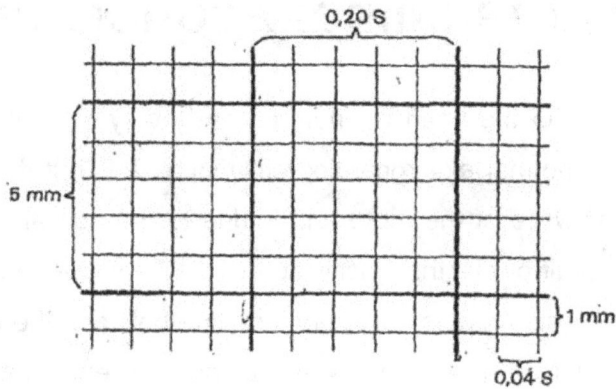

Fig 2.2 Electrocardiogram paper

In electrocardiography, measures vertically, ie upwards or downwards, which indicate the height and depth of the waves, are expressed in millimeters, but measures in respect horizontal, representing the width of the waves, are expressed in fractions of seconds. It follows that each little picture small, equivalent to 0.04 s. This time value is given by the speed with which the paper to join the plot, which is usually 25mm per second, meaning that in a second paper covers 25mm, or 5 pictures of the big move: Therefore, a picture of the great amounts to a fifth of a second (0.20 s) and how each box has five major divisions every small little picture is equivalent to a fifth of 0.20 (0.04 s).

Study of the derivations

The derivation is the place or location of the body where the electrodes are placed to collect the electrocardiographic tracing.

At the beginning of the electrocardiography, only three leads were used, they were the standard or classic known as DI, DII and DIII are bipolar leads, ie, they are become using two electrodes, positive or negative browser and or indifferent, these three leads are those that constitute celebrate Einthoven triangle shown in fig. 2.3 and summarized in Table 2.1

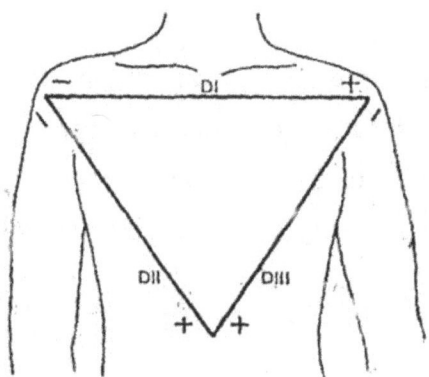

20

Fig 2.3 Representation of the Einthoven triangle with the three standard leads, DI, DII and DIII which constitute the three sides of an equilateral triangle.

Derivation	Probing electrode (+)	Neutral electrode (-)
I	Left arm	Right arm
II	Left Leg	Right arm
III	Left Leg	Left arm

It is important to point out that, when preparing an electrocardiogram, four electrodes are placed on the patient: two on the forearms and two of the legs. This arrangement differs greatly from what is shown n figure 2.3, but what is really happening is that the electrode that is placed on the right leg is introduced into the circuit only to balance the circuit. In particular, that electrode provides a ground. Although the electrodes are placed at the level of the wrists and ankles for ease of application, what the electrodes catch is the electric potential coming out of the member under study. For that reason, the electrodes are schematically placed at the level of the left shoulder and the low and central portions of the abdomen, since the electric potential that goes in the on both lower limbs is essentially the same that shows up on the lower abdomen. In fact, one may interchange the leg electrodes without producing any changes. More. One could place leg electrodes on a single leg, as in the case of amputations, burns or other problems without any changes in the traces.

Soon enough, the need to explore the electrical phenomenon produced by the heart from separate angles, in order to a better understanding of the orientation of electrical forces; the precordial derivations were created in this way, when the electrodes are placed on the patient's chest. These derivations are single-pole. That means, only the positive or probing electrode is used.

Later, E. Godberger created the single-pole derivations of limbs aVR, aVL and VF. These acronyms are explained later.

Currently, an electrocardiogram consists of 12 derivations, including 6 limb derivations DI, DIL, DIII, aVR, aVL and aVF, plus 6 precordial derivations labeled with the letter V (voltage), namely: V1, V2, V3, V4, V5 and V6.

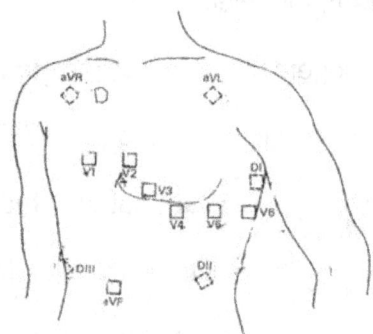

Fig 2.4 Schematic representation of derivations

The anatomical regions on which the potentials of single-pole derivations are detected are listed below:

aVR: at the right shoulder level.

aVL: at the left shoulder lever.

aVF: at the left foot level.

VI: on the fourth rib space, to the right of the sternum.

V2: on the fourth rib space, to the left right of the sternum.

V3: on a location equidistant from both V2 and V4.

V4: on the fifth rib space, on the median clavicular line.

V5: on the fifth rib space, on the anterior maxillary line.

V6: on the fifth rib space, on the median maxillary line.

It is imperative for the student of electrocardiography to know exactly the location of every single derivation; that is easy when the derivations are single-pole, meaning that the only probing pole is used, because these are represented at the same location where the derivation is done; this is not the case with bipolar or standard derivations DI, DII and DIII, in which the positive, probe electrode is influenced by a negative electrode and, in order to represent them through a single electrode (in this case the positive electrode), its position will have to be changed somewhat; to do this, the three-axe Bailey reference system must be used, which consists of displacing the three sides of the Einthoven triangle in order to make the central point of each derivation coincide with the a point located on the center of the triangle (Fig. 2.5).

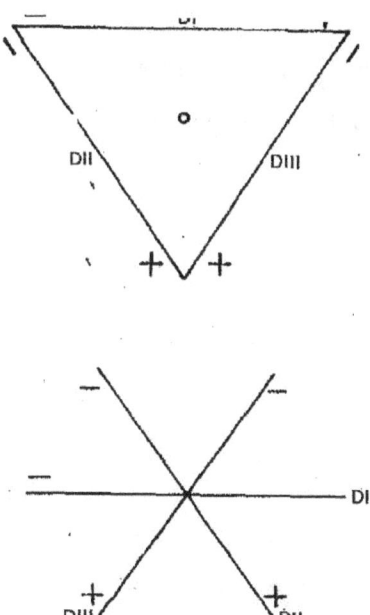

Fig. 2.5 The Einthoven triangle and the three-axe reference system, derived from the latter.

In the three-axe system, the DI positive electrode is placed on the left, towards the axillary region, much like the V6 location. DII is registered with the positive electrode towards the lower left hemiabdomen, while the DIII positive electrode is located towards the right lower hemiabdomen, all in the direction of the center of the thorax, as shown in figure 2.4.

When studying derivations, it is important to know from which angle they sense the process of Electrical activation of the heart, in order to be able to accurately determine the spatial orientation of the of vectors, because, as is known, activation waves that move getting closer to a derivation produce positive waves on the path and vice versa; Therefore, we can conclude that: V5, V6, DI and aVL are left derivations, i.e., they explore the heart electrical activity from the left side; V1 and V2 are right precordial because they explore the heart electrical activity from right ventricle; aVR makes it up and to the right, down and to the right, and aVF, DII DILI and DILI explore the posterior side of the heart, since they sense the potentials that are distributed to the lower portion of the body and as is known, the back of the heart is more likely posteroinferior (it is called diaphragmatic because it rests on the diaphragm).

The front face of the heart is studied by the precordial derivations (VI, V2, and V3 to the right) And V4, V5, and V6 (toward the left anterolateral portion).

The electrical activation of the heart can produce a completely different morphology in the traces, depending on which place or derivation where the process of activation (fig. 2.6) is picked up

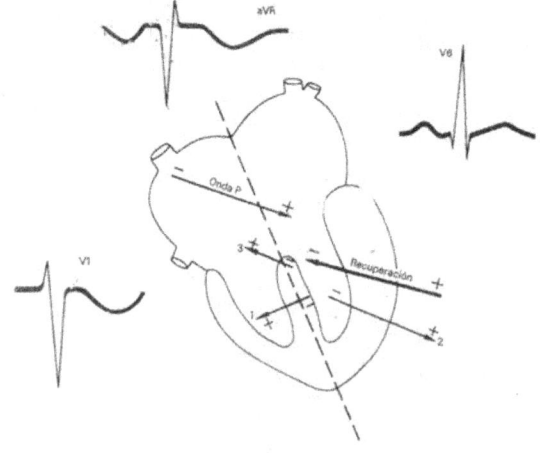

2.6. Different morphologies of electrocardiogram waves in relation to the derivation

Figure 2.6 shows how a normal activation produces complexes of different morphology depending on where the activation process is picked up; an electrode located upwards and to the right, such as aVR, picks up the auricular vector or P wave as a negative wave because this vector is moving away from the electrode; as regards the QRS complex, the first activation vector, which corresponds to the septum, will not be picked up because its orientation is fully perpendicular to the line of derivation (interrupted line); vector 2 is picked up as a strongly negative wave because it, too, is moving away from the electrode; and; lastly, remnant vector produces on this derivation a small final positivity. As for the wave of recovery (T-wave) also is also marked negative in this derivation because, in fact the aVR derivation mo in this is known as the derivation of negativities, because usually all there is negative: the P wave, the QRS complex and the T wave.

If the same the same activation process is registered with an electrode on the right, such as V1, the vector P may not be picked up well because it is almost perpendicular to the line of this derivation (fig. 2.6); as regards to the QRS complex, a small positive wave is picked up first; this done by activating the septum, whose wave moves towards this electrode and the right ventricular wall activation is then added. Lastly, a sharply negative wave is produced, which is caused by vector 2, which is directed to the left; vector 3 is not picked up due to its orientation, which is upwards and back, because, in all cases, it contributes to emphasize more the negativity of 2 vector. The recovery wave is also entered as a negative wave. The right precordial derivations effectively have these features: the QRS complex begins with a small positive wave and continues with a predominantly negative wave.

If the derivation under study is on the left (V6, V5, DI), the complex morphology is quite different: positive P-waves, complex QRS begins with a small negative wave (the Q wave) due to septum activation, which is followed by a strongly positive wave, since vector 2 comes closer to the electrode that is to the left. Lastly, the vector remnant marks a small negative wave.

The recovery wave in this case (the T wave) is positive; we must remember that the T wave should normally follow the main deflection of the QRS complex. The left derivations, therefore, have these general characteristics: they start with a small negativity and are predominantly positive.

These morphological concepts of right and left derivations are fundamental, above all when assessing the morphology of the patterns in the precordial series.

Measurements of interest in electrocardiography

A number of aspects must be determined in every electrocardiogram. A logical pre-stablished order must be followed, in order not to miss any derivation of importance in the diagnostic. These aspects are: rhythm, heart rate, P-wave, PR interval, QRS complex (orientation or electrical axis, duration or width and voltage or height,), ST segment and T wave.

Rhythm

The first determination to be performed in any electrocardiogram is whether the rate is sinusoidal. A sinusoidal rhythm is identified in an electrocardiogram whenever every complex QRS is preceded by its corresponding P wave; therefore there is equal number of P waves to QRS complexes. One must also see whether or not the distance since the start of the P wave to the QRS complex, which is called the PR interval or Ligature is always the same, which means that activation comes out in the normal form from the sinusoidal node and activates the auricles (P waves), traversed the AV node and the His bundle (the PR segment) and finally the ventricles (fig. 2.7)

When the above is not fulfilled, one is dealing with of heart rhythm disorder, or arrhythmia.

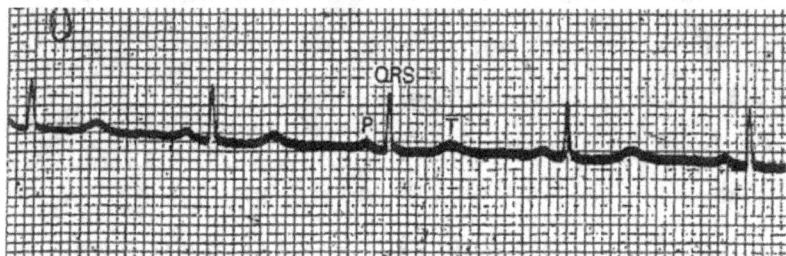

Fig 2.7 sinus rhythm. Observe that each QRS complex is preceded by its PR and P wave is equal (heart rate 15002075)

Heart rate

To determine the number of heart beats per minute: this is done by dividing 1 500 between the number of small squares between two successive QRS complexes.

1500, a constant. In a 1 s paper, paper will move 25 small squared (25 mm), therefore in 1 min will travel 1500 mm. that is 25 x 60. If for example, there are 20 small squared between a QRS complex and the next QRS complex, which is 1 min, there will be 1 500/20 = 75, which is the heart rate (fig. 2.7).

Normal heart rate for an adult is between 60 to 100 beats per minute.

The P Wave

In any electrocardiogram, it is of paramount importance to identify the P wave, which, as he has been said, is the first wave resulting from electrical activation of auricles; and once identified, one must carefully study its morphology. The most suitable derivation to identify the P wave is DII, because of the agreement with the normal inclination of the wave of activation (down and to the left), it comes close to such derivation and, therefore, reaches its highest voltage in there.

The Normal P wave is a thick trace wave and round outline. Its height is generally below 2.5 mm (fig 2.8A).

When auricular hypertrophy exists, the P-wave voltage changes and, above all, its morphology; of changes. In this way, if hypertrophy is on the right auricle, the P wave becomes symmetrical and sharp, as well as higher (fig 2.8b). In this case the P axis turns somewhat to the right, the pulmonary P-waves are better identified in DII, DII and aVF, as well as in the right precordial derivations VI and V2.

When hypertrophy is on the left auricle, the P-wave adopts a different morphology. It becomes wider, is flattens at its peak, and often presents a notch, which is the so-called mitral P wave, that because the P vector leans to the left is, it is seen best in DI and DII, as well as in the V4, V5 and V.6 left precordial derivations (fig. 2.8 c).

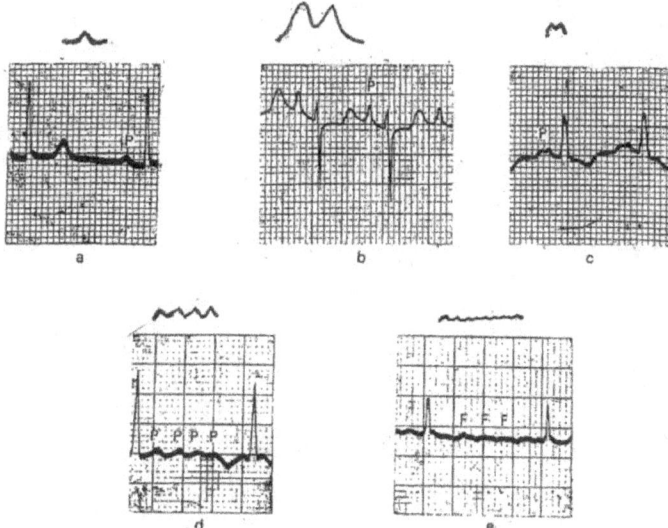

Fig 2.8 The normal P wave; b, pulmonary; c, mitral; d, saw tooth (P-wave or flutter handset); e, atrial fibrillation (waves F)

The PR interval

As been said before, the PR interval is the period of time that goes from the beginning of the P wave to the beginning of the QRS complex, its measurement, therefore includes: the duration of the wave P (the atrial electrical) and the PR segment, which as you know is the time that it takes for the electrical activation to traverse the ventricular auricular node and the His bundle; However, the measurement is always performed jointly to simplify reading because an alteration in the duration of the PR interval always occurs, which is due to the time that it takes the stimulus in traversing the node AV (PR segment) (fig. 2.9)

The normal duration of the PR interval is variable according to the heart rate, since the PR interval frequency tends to shorten at higher frequencies, but in general terms, maximum normal limits may be accepted between 0.20 s and up to 0.16 s in the child, provided that heart rate is within normal limits.

When PR interval is elongated or variable, there is a difficulty in the conduction of the electric stimulus through the AV node, which is referred to as AV block and according to the degree of difficulty in the conduction, may be first, second or third grade.

When the PR interval is very shortened, (in fact there is no PR segment) one speaks of the existence of pre-excitation syndrome or Wolff-Parkinson-White (fig. 2.9) all of which will be dealt with in the Chapter on disorders of the heartbeat.

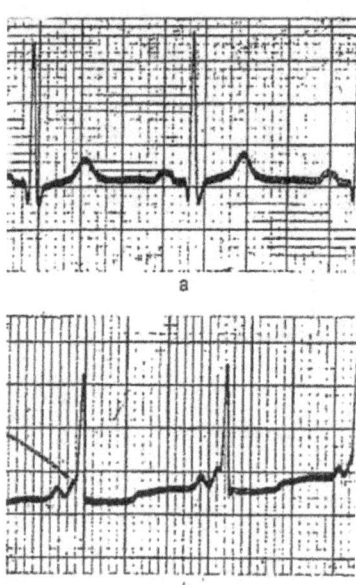

Fig. 2.9 The PR interval: a, normal; b, Wolff-Parkinson-White syndrome. There is no PR segment.

The Median electric axis

The median electrical axis of the QRS complex is the orientation in the front vector 2 of the ventricular activation, which, as seen before, is the resultant vector of activation power of both ventricles. This vector must normally be oriented downward and to the left, due to the fact that, since because wall of the left ventricle is thicker, with the result that are predominant, electrical forces are predominant.

If the precordial region is divided into four quadrants and circumference is drawn around it, the electric axis will normally be on the left lower quadrant (fig. 2.10), i.e. between 0 and 90 (in electrocardiography the two lower quadrants have positive values, while the top quadrants have negative values).

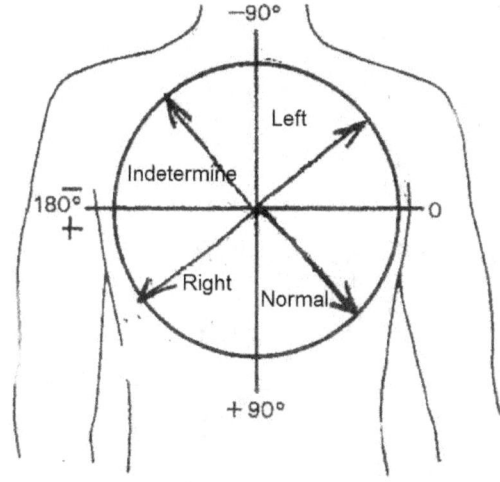

Fig. 2.10 Schematic division of precordial region in quadrant's.

When the electric axis is in the right lower quadrant, i.e. between 90 and 180°, is a right axis deviation is said to exist.

When the electrical axis occupies the left upper quadrant, i.e. between 0 and - 90 °, there is a left axial derivation.

Finally, when the axis occupies the upper right quadrant, is in a position, this is an indeterminate position, between -90 ° and 180 °.

Classically, for the determination of the orientation of the electric front axis, standard derivations DI and DIII are used only, although occasionally, as seen later, one must aide oneself by using the DII derivation.

The fact that derivations referrals DI and DIII are so useful in this determination is due to the fact that both study the electrical potential produced by the heart from opposite angles. It may be remembered that DI is a derivation located the left side, while DIII is located downward and to the right. It is important to remember this location as a memory aid, you may use the fact that DI always appears in an electrocardiogram of the left and DIII always appears to the right.

By using this concept, the determination of the orientation of the axis electric is much easier: when the electric is deviated to the left axis, current or wave of activation approaches DI; therefore, this derivation exhibits a QRS pattern of a positive strong prevalence, at the same time that the ORS DIII pattern is predominantly negative, i.e. the positive wave is located in front to the left of the observer (fig 2.1 and 2. 12a).

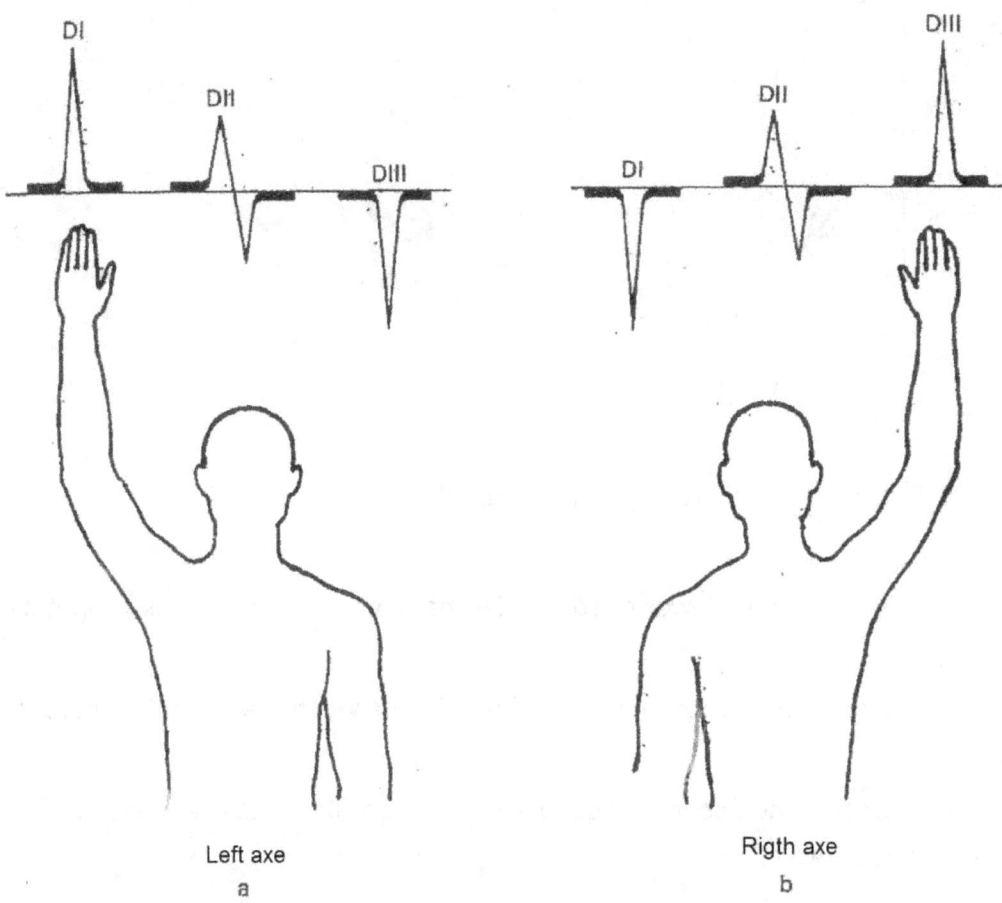

Left axe

a

Rigth axe

b

Fig. 2.11 Scheme that exemplifies the deviation of two QRS electric axes.

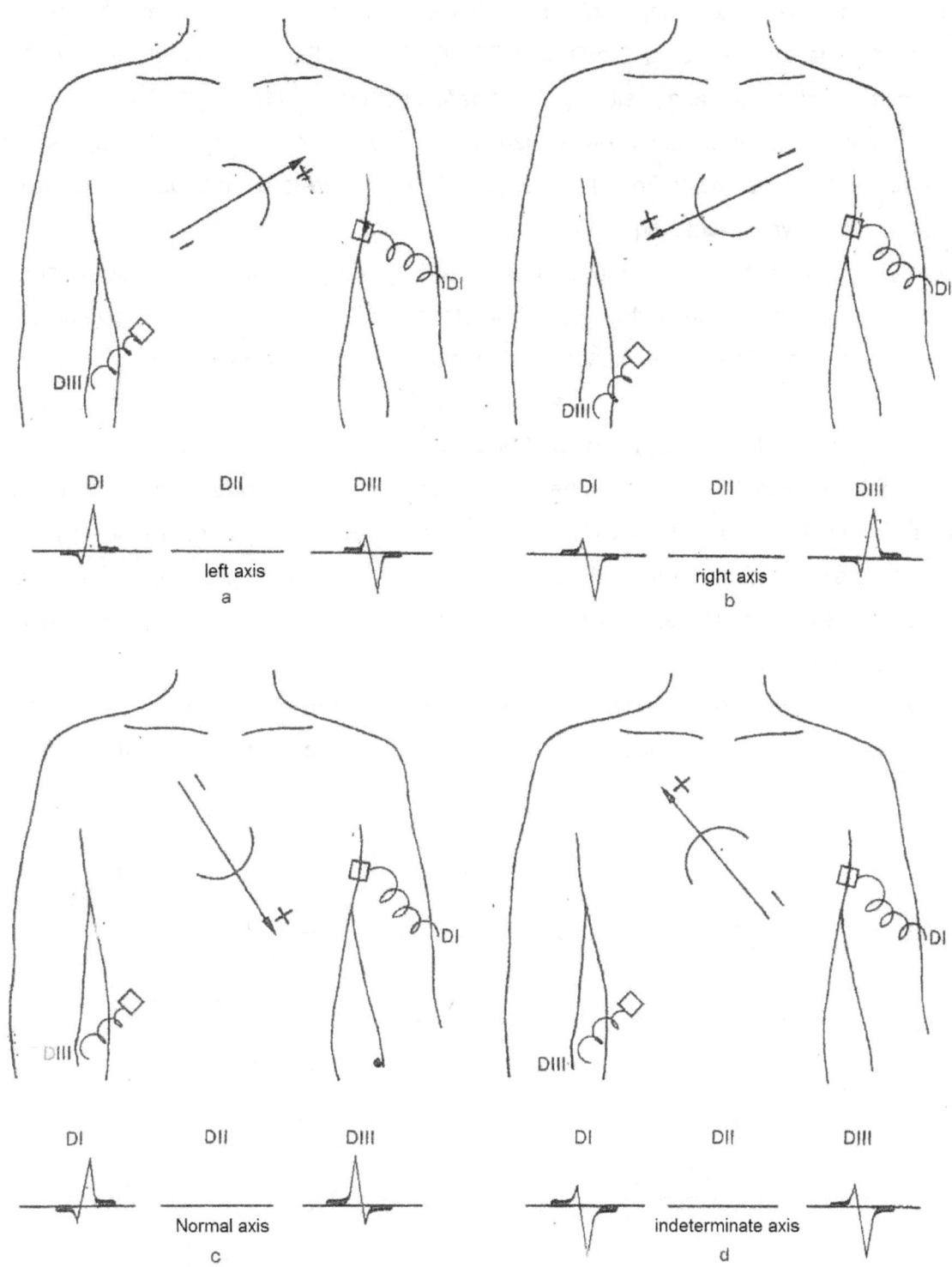

Fig 2.12 Different electrical axis deviations

When this electrical axis in normal position, the inclination of the vector or ventricular activation wave is down and to the left, approaching electrodes DI and DIII, and this makes the QRS patterns predominantly positive both in DI and DIII (fig 2.11 a); that is, in the electric axes that have a normal position there is a positive predominance both in DI and DIII.

If the axes are in an indeterminate position, the activation vector or wave is directed upward and to the right, and moves away from both of DI as DIII. Therefore both derivations exhibit predominantly negative patterns (fig 211a).

It is necessary to clarify that if you analyze electrocardiograms, you will detect that the electric axis is in the normal or indeterminate position, no other another consideration is necessary, the first event is normal and the indeterminate position is always pathological; however, if the axis is oriented to the left or the right, it is important to know whether or not if this deviation is light or marked, since in the first case may not be pathological.

In order to make a determination on whether a deviation is right or left, one must avail oneself of the DII-derivation. If DII exhibits a QRS pattern with a clearly predominantly positivity, the deviation of the axis is not very marked, However, if the QRS pattern appearing in DII is a small voltage, isodiphasic, or negative, the deviation is marked and much more so with increasing negativity in the pattern DII.

The above is also the same on deviated to that right in those deviated to the left, because, as shown in Figure 2.13, negative values of DII increase as the vector leans more to the right or to the left.

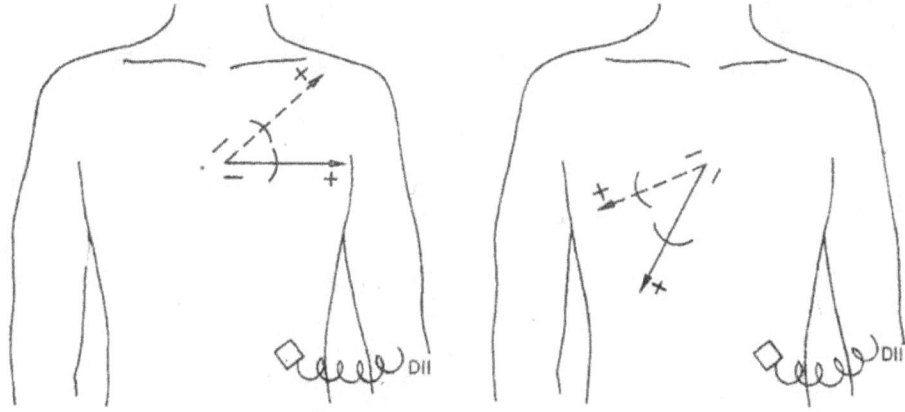

Fig 2.13 A schematic representation from the DII electric field derivation on the slightly or greatly deviated axis, either to the left and to the right.

One last consideration is needed in relation to the electrical axis, and is the not uncommon case, in which in one of the derivations DI or DII, undefined pattern appears, i.e. isodiphasic or equal to zero; in reality, these axes are the best defined, because, when the pattern isodiphasic or equal to zero in one of these derivations, it means that the electric axis is perpendicular to the line of the derivation; so, if the pattern is isodiphasic on DI, the axis can amount to 90° or -90°.

If the pattern is isodiphasic on DII, the shaft would be +30° or -150°, but it is necessary to specify well, because in both cases the shaft may be normal or extremely pathological.

If this case occurs, proceed as follows:

1. When the QRS pattern in the derivation DI or DIII is isodiphasic or equal to zero, deemed this pattern is equal to what is shown on the opposite branch.

2. If DI shows an isodiphasic pattern and DIII is positive, both will therefore be considered positive, in this case the axis is normal, 90°.

3. If DI has an isodiphasic pattern and DIII exhibits a predominantly negative pattern, both will be considered negative and in this case the axis is indeterminate, - 90°.

4. If DIII has an isodiphasic pattern and the pattern of DI is positive, both will be considered positive as you positive and the axis in this case is normal, +30°.

5. If DIII has an isodiphasic pattern and the pattern of DI is predominantly negative, both will be considered negative and, in the case, the axis is undetermined -150°,

6. If both patterns, both of the derivation DI as that of DIII were isodiphasic (a rare occurrence), the axis is considered to be in the normal position; usually in these cases the patterns are isodiphasic in all members' derivations and are due to a completely circular vector loop.

An electric axis that is much towards the left or the right, indicates a frank predominance of electric forces to the respective side, and therefore may suggest a ventricular hypertrophy in most cases, but not necessarily; so for example or full fascicular or bunch Branch blocks, and heart attacks can produce strong deviations of the electric axis, while also, there may be ventricular hypertrophy that does not deviate the! Electric axis. There may also be deviations of the axis to the opposite side, as will be seen in chapter 4, i.e. that electric axe deviations always will have to be evaluated them in conjunction with the rest of the alterations that appear on the trace.

Electric Position

The electric position, as well as electric axis position, is an indicator of orientation at the front plane of the forces of the QRS activation.

The procedure most often used to determine the electrical position, is to check the morphology of the QRS complexes present in the aVL, and aVF derivations; as is known, the aVL derivation explores the heart from the upper left chest, while aVF doe same from the lower portion.

As one would logically assume, the electric horizontal position is one that exhibits predominantly positive QRS patterns in the aVL derivation, while of small or negative voltages on the aVF derivation; the vertical electric positions, on the contrary, show strongly positive QRS complex in the aVF derivation, but show a weak or no positivity on aVL;, lastly hearts in intermediate electrical position show positive predominance of QRS patterns both on aVL and aVF.

Under normal conditions, in a heart that is considered an intermediate position because it is not turned to one side or another, the ventricles are oriented in the following way: the right, to the right and forward; the left, to the left, before and below; for that reason, hearts in an intermediate position show predominantly positive QRS patterns (similar to what shows in the V5 and V6) derivations and representative of the left ventricle show both on the aVL and aVF derivations (Fig. 2.14.a)

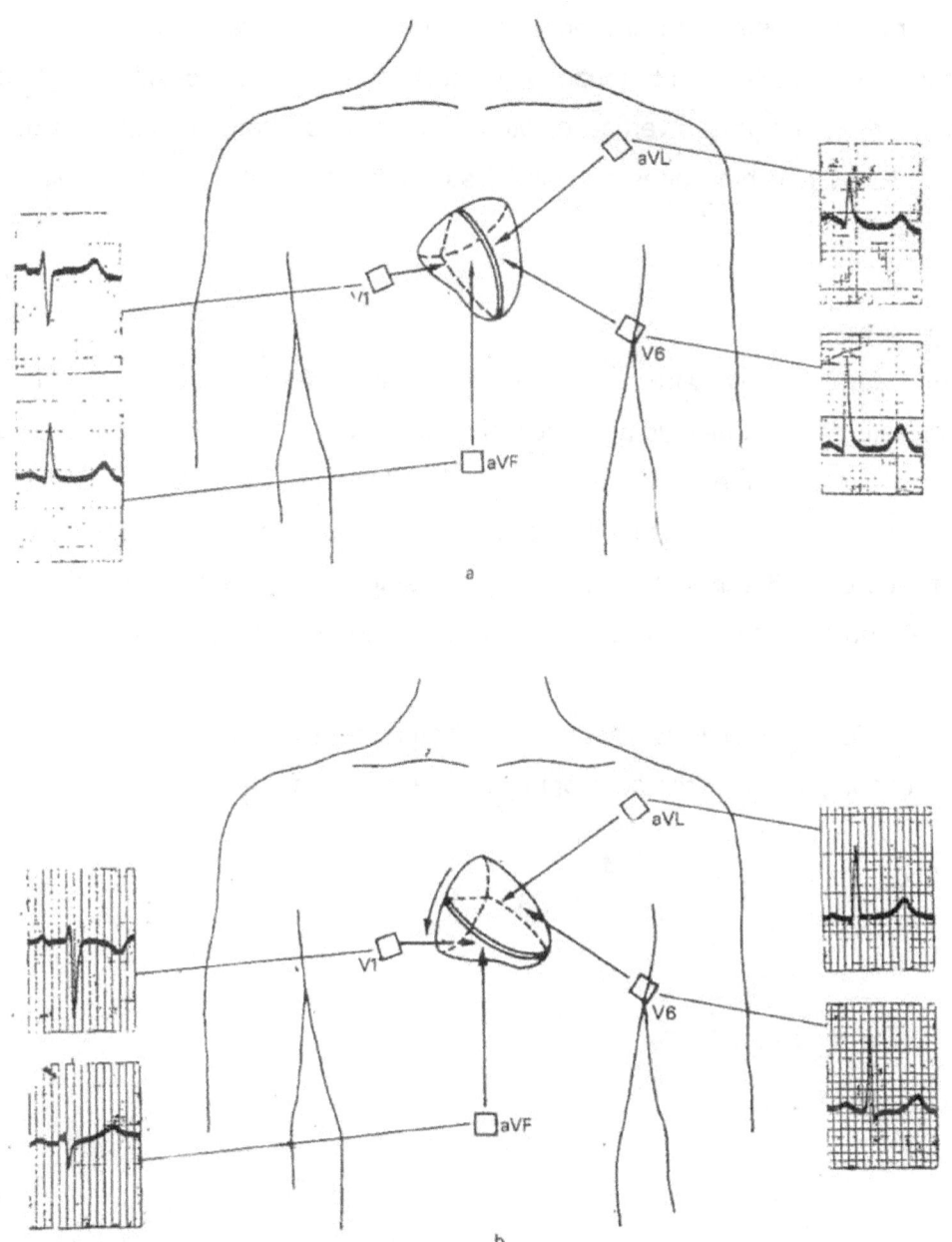

Fig 2.14 Electric position electric: a, intermediate; b, horizontal and c, vertical.

When the heart is rotated around its longitudinal axis and the left ventricle is close to the top and front, predominantly positive QRS patterns appear on the aVL derivation (fig. 2.14 b); on the other hand, when the rotation is such that the main muscle mass or free wall of left ventricular left rests on the diaphragm, QRS patterns are predominantly positive, similar to what shows on V5 and V6, appear in the aVF derivation, while QRS patters on aVL show a low voltage or are negative (fig. 2.14 c).

In conclusion, the patterns of the left ventricle morphology, often become visible on the DI and aVL deviations, in those hearts that are in a horizontal electric or intermediate position, and on DII, DIII and aVF, the hearts which have a vertical electric position. This is important in the study of the ventricular hypertrophy and blockades of branch, as will be seen at the end of related chapters.

.

QRD complex Duration or width

This is a measurement taken horizontally from the beginning of the QRS complex to completion, and indicates the time lasting for the electric activation of ventricles. Normally, it can take up to 0.10 s (two squares and a half) in the adult and up to 0.08 s (two small squares) in children; These are maximum figures, that is to say that it is rare to see electrocardiograms with a 0 0.1 QRS duration in an adult s or 0.08 s in a child, that are non-pathological. The minimum figures are of no interest, there is no any pathology because the QRS complex is very narrow.

Usually, the QRS complex length or width of is stretched when there is a difficulty or disorder in electric intraventricular conduction, as in the case of bundle branch locks.

QRS complex wave voltage of height

The QRS complex may exhibit low or high wave voltage; low voltage can be seen in one series of very different processes interfering with electric conduction, while the high voltage is one of the most important alterations in ventricular hypertrophy. Next, we analyze the criteria utilized when dealing with diagnostics of low or high voltage.

Low QRS complex voltage

The QRS complex is said to be of low voltage, when the arithmetical sum of the positive and negative waves of the QRS complex does not exceed 5 mm in any of three derivations (fig. 2.1 5) standard. It is necessary to point out that the small complex must be present in the three derivations, because no diagnostic is possible if the measurement just given is exceeded in any derivation.

A low voltage in the QRS complex is seen mostly on processes that interfere with electric conduction, such as acute myocarditis, myxedema or hypothyroidism, large overflow pericarditis pulmonary emphysema, obesity, etc.

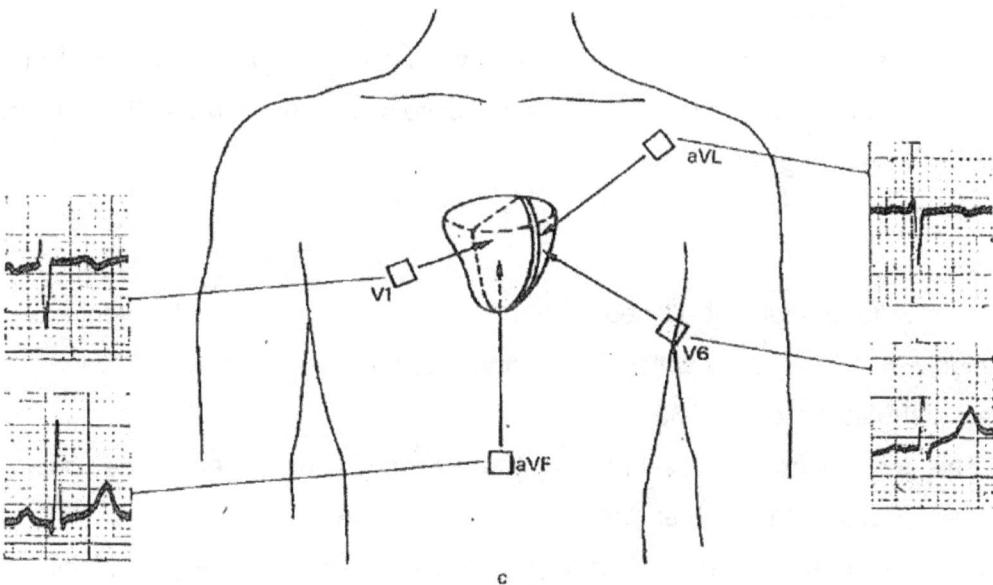

Fig. 2.15 A Low voltage QRS complex, the arithmetic sum of positive and negative waves of the complex QRS does not exceed 5 mm in any of three standard derivations. As it usually occurs, the T waves are also flattened.

<u>High QRS complex voltage</u>

The high voltage of the QRS complex can be seen when looking at the high-altitude or depth of the QRS complex in standard derivations; However, these derivations, no systematic measurements of height or depth of waves is taken, because, the high voltage of the complex QRS is one of the more important data in the diagnosis of the ventricular hypertrophy, where voltage measurements need to be taken, because such measurements are of particular interest, that explore the heart from the right or the left or from the left side; so for example, the following are important:

For the right ventricle

1. The VI R wave. This voltage must not exceed 10 mm, except for children under two years of age. Usually this derivation must be predominantly negative; just dominate the wavelength R over S, i.e., the ratio. R/S > 1 is abnormal.
2. The aVR R wave. Normally the QRS complex in the aVR derivation should be predominantly negative; If this pattern is isodiphasic or predominantly positive, it is pathological, except in children below one month of age.
3. The aVL S wave. This is a derivation located to the left; when greatly negative it indicates that there are important electrical forces inclined toward the opposite side. A wave More than 10 mm of depth in aVL is usually pathological.

For the left ventricle:

1. The V6 R wave. Its voltage shall not exceed 25 mm, if it is higher, suggests left ventricular hypertrophy; commonly this V6 R-wave voltage adds depth of V1 S wave of (Sokolow index), and this measurement should not exceed 35 mm.
2 The V2 S wave. This Is considered representative of the left ventricle and when the depth is more than 25mm, it suggests ventricle hypertrophy.
3. The aVL R wave. It is considered normal up to 13 mm, if this measurement is higher, it suggests left ventricular hypertrophy.

The ST-segment

After the ventricles are electrically activated, a thick trace appears, which occupies the isloelectric line, also known as the ST-segment, which must be at the same level! of its counterpart of the opposite side (the RT segment). The ST-segment coincides with the mechanical work (ventricle contraction) and separates the electrical activation complex (QRS) from the recovery or T wave.

When interpreting an electrocardiogram, the level differences of the isoelectric line segment ST are important. The pathologies that may produce segment T level variations are several; level differences may be positive or negative and, in either case, the level difference must be evaluated jointly with the accompanying T wave. Level differences must be greater and 1 mm.

A positive segment ST level difference with a high, positive T wave suggests vagotomy; a flattened T wave suggests pericarditis and a strongly inverted T wave suggests acute myocardium infarction (fig 2 16 a).

A negative segment ST level difference with a highly positive T wave suggests subendocardiac ischemia; a normal R wave suggests digitalis impregnation, all the more so if the ST segment is in the shape of a vat. An inverted T wave suggests a ventricular overload (fig 2.16b).

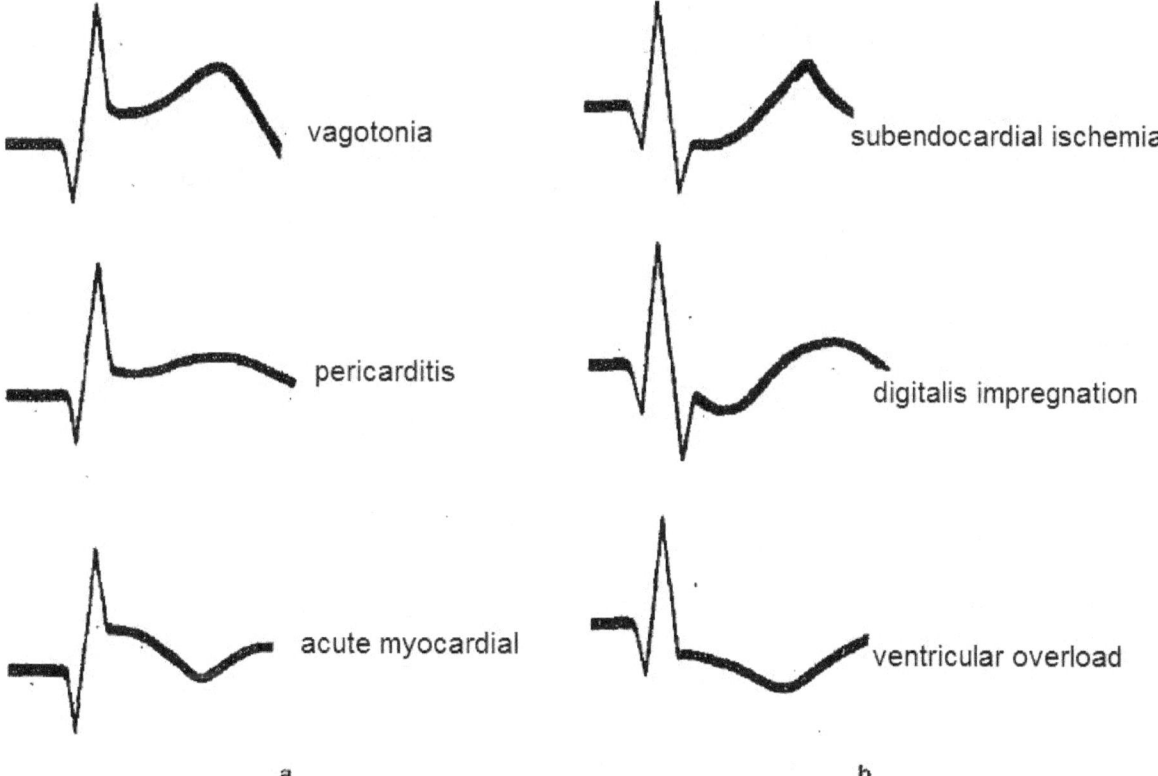

vagotonia

subendocardial ischemia

pericarditis

digitalis impregnation

acute myocardial

ventricular overload

a

b

Fig 2.16b   ST segment level differences: a, positive level differences: b, negative level differences.

The alterations mentioned above suggest these pathologies, but must be examined clinically, because an electrocardiogram is a complementary examination that must be evaluated in the light of clinical manifestations.

<u>The T wave</u>.

As was said before, this is the ventricular recovery wave; it is slow, traces thick strokes is and rounded contours.

The T wave must be positive in all derivations except aVR derivations and VI, where the T wave is usually negative and, occasionally, the DIII derivation.

In general, the T wave orientation must match the orientation of the QRS to complex that it accompanies, i.e. if the QRS complex is predominantly positive, the T wave should also be positive; this aspect is of great importance when evaluating a negative T wave.

In children, as will be explained in chapter 7, the T wave can be inverted in the right precordial series, including V4 and this does not mean a disease if the trace of other alterations is missing. (persistence of a youth pattern).

3 Cardiac rhythm disturbances

Normally the electrical impulse is generated without usual nodule located in the upper part of the handset right, near mouth of the superior deep vein; this is the nodule which governs the activity of the heart, and for this reason is called pacemaker.

As you remember, the electric impulse sinus is driven through of bundles internodal, anterior, middle and posterior to the AV node currently known as the region of the union, located at the bottom of the handset right, close of the interatrial septum.

After passing through the region of the union stimulus arrives to the bundle of his and this happens to the ventricular walls and septum, through a system trifascicular right branch of the bundle of his and two fascicles of the left, anterior and posterior branch; the ramifications of this trifascicular arborizations of Purkinje system were distributed by the ventricles endocardial surface and the septum to convey the electrical impulse to these areas.

Classification of arrhythmias

Arrhythmias can be classified in different ways, then the classification that takes into account both the alterations in the formation of the impulse and those that arise in the conduct of this is synthesized in a box.

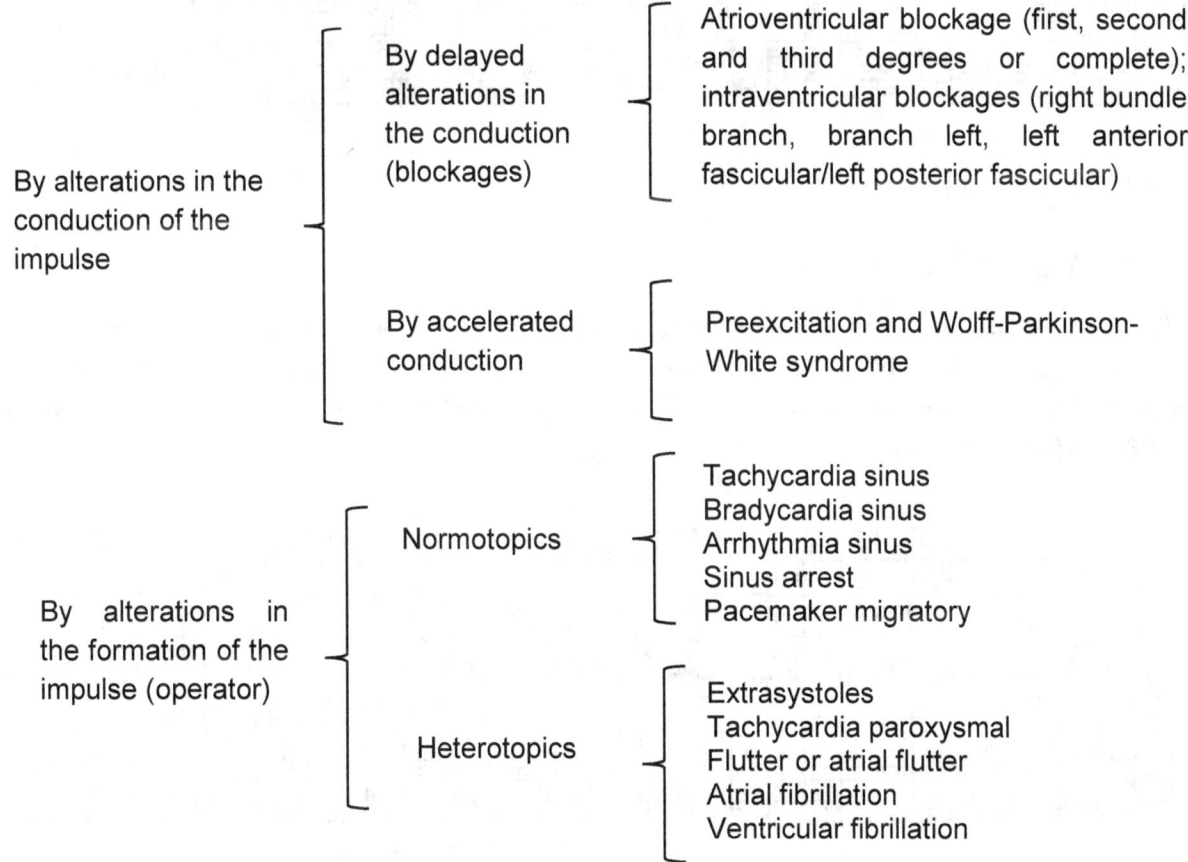

41

Atrial fibrillation ventricular fibrillation arrhythmias by alterations in the formation of the impulse (Automation)

Normotopics Arrhythmias

In this type of arrhythmia the altered stimulus generated in the sinus node.

Tachycardia sinus

in this alteration the stimulus usually originated in the nodule sinus is reiterated an often exaggerated, exceeding 100 beats per minute; from the electrocardiographic point of view, this tachycardia is characterized, first, because the heart rate is rarely going more beyond 160 beats per minute; also the wavelength P is always recognizable and normal characteristics, like the rest of the waves of the path.

The only alteration is the shortening of the space diastolic or TP: i.e. space which goes from the T wave to the P-wave of the next complex, than in these houses is considerably shortened or is inexistence, and wave P occurs nearly over I to the previous complex T wave (Fig 3.1),

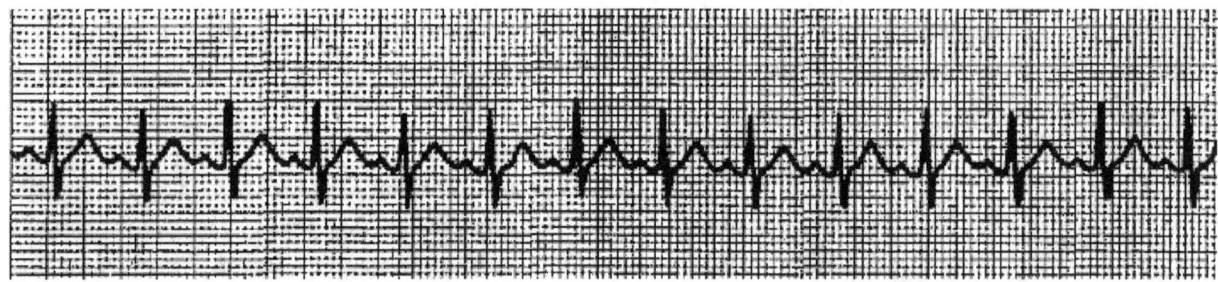

Fig 3.1 Tachycardia sinus

Sinus bradycardia

As in the previous case, the stimulus usually originates in the sinus node, but it does so at a very slow rate, less than 60 beats per minute. From the point of view ECG sinus bradycardia is characterized because all the waves of the path are normal, only diastolic TP this greatly elongated space (fig: 3.2).

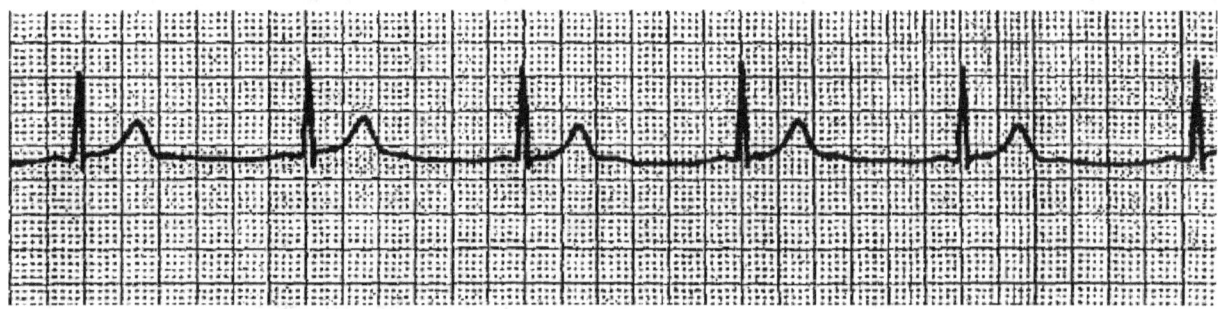

Fig 3.2 Bradycardia sinus

Arrhythmia sinus

The stimulus does also in the sinus node, but it reiterates at time intervals that are unequal. From the electrocardiographic point of view, this arrhythmia is characterized because the QRS complexes are not equally spaced. Diagnose the difference must be greater than 0.12 mm (3 squares) in a complex to the following and said to be step; It has no interest from the point of view clinical (fig.3.3).

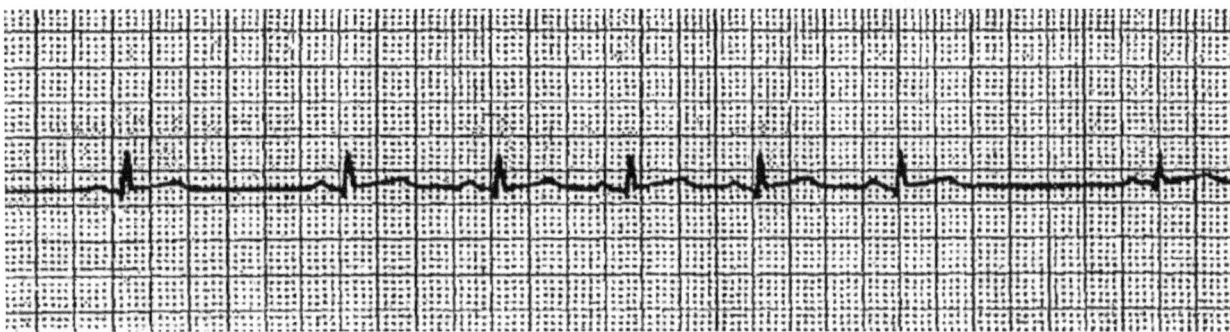

Fig 3.3. Arrhythmia sinus.

Sinus arrest

Consists in the lack of generation of a stimulus within the sinus rhythm. From the point of view of electrocardiographic is characterized by the absence of a heartbeat by what appears a pause diastolic extended between two normal heartbeats; this pause interval is the corresponding to the two normal cycles or slightly less (fig. 3.4).

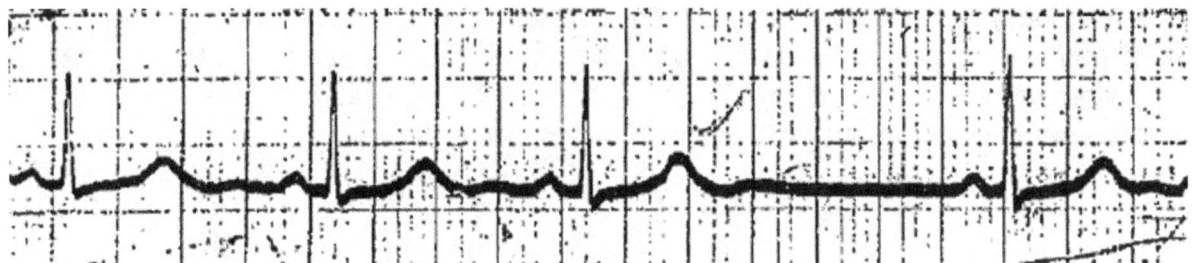

Fig 3.4 stopping sinus after the third complex there is a pause that spans the length of two cycles.

Pacemaker migratory

Immigration the pacemaker stimuli is not always generated at the same site, from the point of view of electrocardiographic, characterized because in a same derivation, P-waves are of variable morphology, even some of it can be negative, since the stimulus can come from the AV node, activating the Atria as retrograde (from bottom-up); in this case, logically there is a component Heterotopic (fig. 3.5).

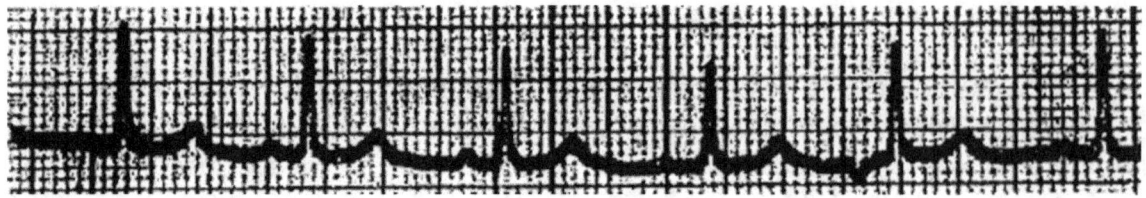

Fig 3.5 immigration pacemaker. P-wave morphologic difference note in different complexes. The fifth beat is a stimulus nodal or union.

Heterotopies Arrhythms

In this type of arrhythmia the stimulus is generated outside sinus, from secondary or tertiary centers (ectopic focus) capable of generating stimuli.

Ectopic beats

Are one of the arrhythmias more frequent; they can be defined as premature cardiac contractions originating from an ectopic focus namely; out of the sinus node

the ectopic beat are recognized easily in the path because extrasystole contraction comes in the base rhythm, i.e., this more next to the above and usually is followed by elongated paused, call pause post extrasystoles or compensatory pause.

The morphology of the QRS complex extrasystoles can be more or less distorted according to the site where originated the abnormal heartbeat; If the stimulation was born in the ventricle, the QRS complex to which it gives rise is wide and deformed (fig 3.6a), but if the extrasystole originated above the ventricles (nodule to V of the bundle of His). When the stimulus is distributed in the normal way by the ventricles the QRS complex feature is normal, although it may differ slightly from the base complex. The ectopic beats may be isolated, grouped in the form of salutes or appear with certain rhythmicity, for example, a normal contraction and an extra systolic and so on, which is called bigeminal rhythm (fig 3.6a); at other times it may appear two normal contractions and an extrasystolic (rhythm trigeminal)

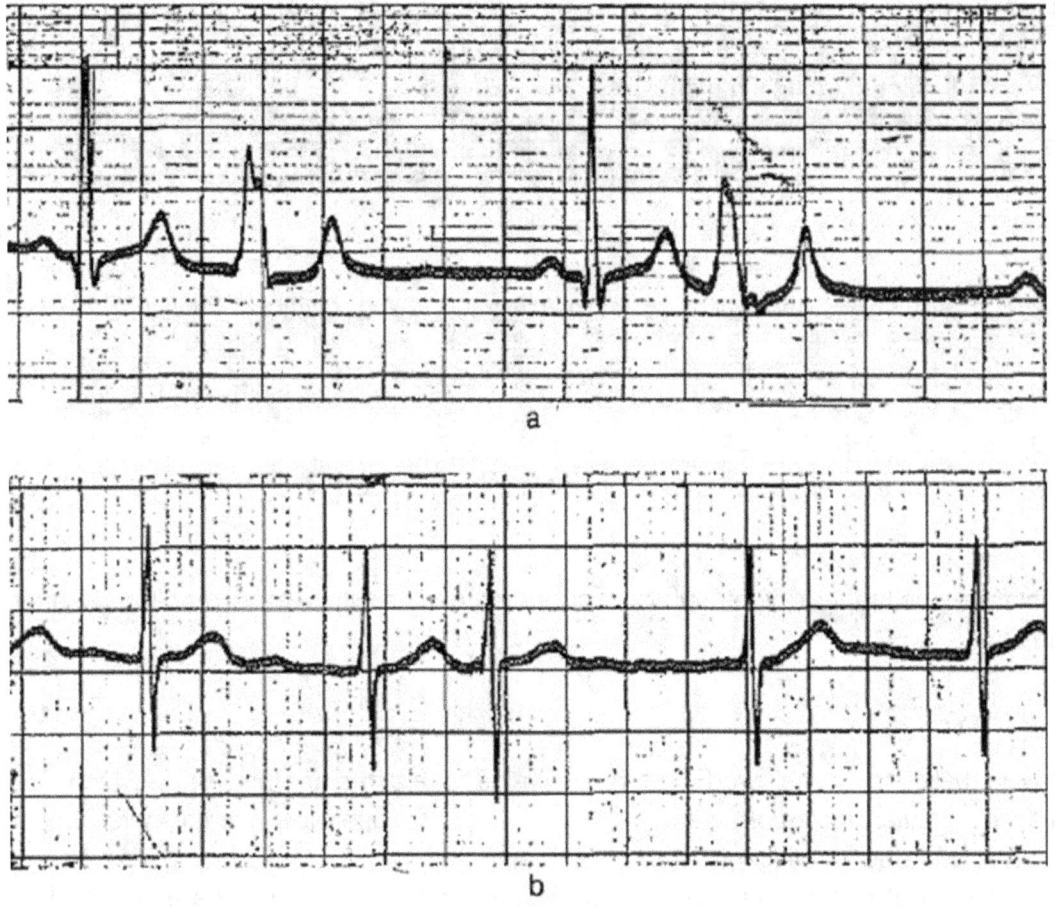

Fig 3.6 Extrasystole: a, ventricular ectopic beats alternating with QRS complexes normal giving a bigeminal rhythm; b, the third complex is an extrasystole supravetricular

Tachycardia functional

Paroxysmal tachycardia can be considered (as an uninterrupted succession of extrasystoles. According to the source site is divided into two large groups: ventricular, when its site of origin below the division of the bundle of His, and supra ventricular, when this site is over the division of the bundle of His.

Paroxysmal ventricular tachycardia (fig. 3.7 to), the morphology of the QRS, as in ventricular ectopic complexes, this very deformed and QRS complexes of great width and conduction disturbances, evidenced by smears of nicks (aberrant complexes), and their waves are produced while tachycardia supraventricular paroxysmal (fig. (3.7 b), QRS complexes retain a more or less normal morphology, however it is difficult to confuse with a sinus tachycardia, first the heavy heart frequency is greater (higher than 160) and normal P waves preceding QRS to the complex cannot be identified.

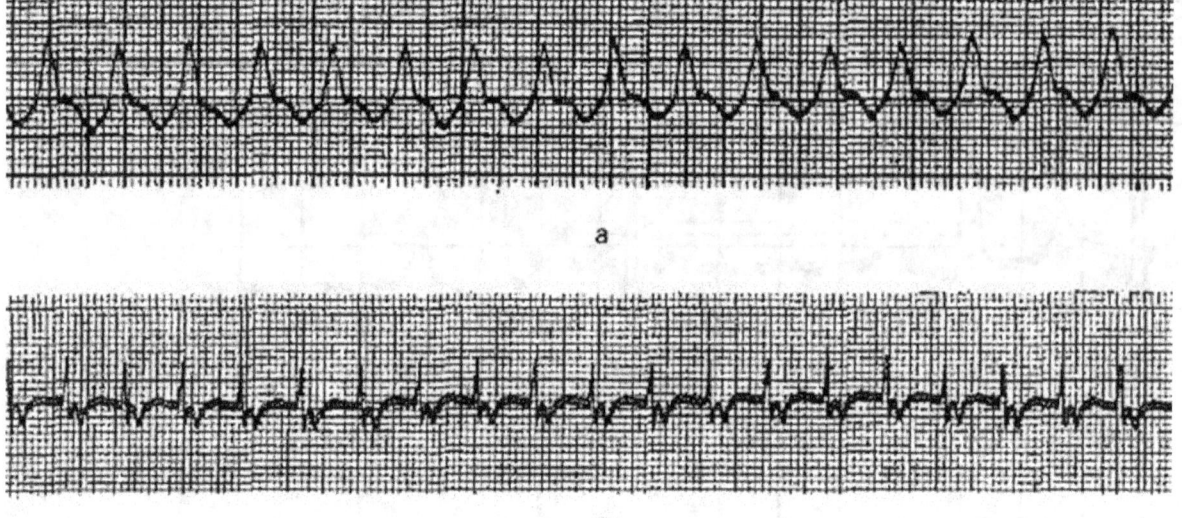

a

b

Fig. 3.7 tachycardia junctional: a, ventricular; b, supraventricular with waves reactionary after the QRS complex.

Flutter or atrial flutter

this arrhythmia is believed to be produced by downloads electric in the Atria, which are distributed in form circular by small areas of tissue and produce new stimuli, with which originated a series of large atrial contractions (200 and 400 per minute), giving rise to the appearance in the path of a large number of P-wave one behind the other, therefore the line isoelectric adopts the appearance of teeth of saw or Festoon. This large number of stimuli headphones the ventricular respond you as regular only each 2, 3 or 4 stimuli headphones, usually in a fixed, therefore the ventricular rate is always regular (fig. 3.8).

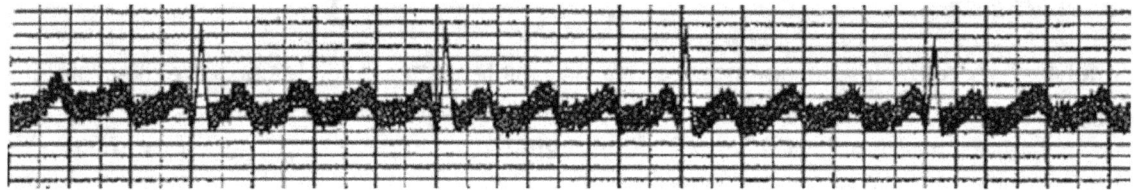

Fig. 3.8 Atrial Flutter.

Atrial fibrillation

Atrial fibrillation the Atria electrical activity is much more messy in this arrhythmia, and is represented by a series of thin plot contractions, which are capable of causing an effective atrial contraction, and the Atria enter a State of tremulation that supports life, under which blood passes from the Atria to the ventricles by gravity.

From the point of view ECG, this arrhythmia is characterized by no P waves but a thin tremulation line isoelectric, which are called F waves or fibrillation and they are being detected better in DII derivations and, above all, V1 and V2. F waves are produced with a very high frequency (between 400 and 800 per minute), and to these small stimulus headphones electric the ventricles respond in very irregular in shape, that is, if the distance is measured between a QRS complex and the next, this will be highly variable (fig. 3.9).

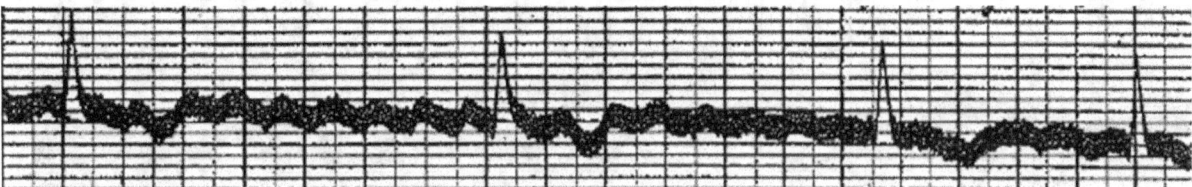

Fig 3.9 Atrial fibrillation.

Ventricular fibrillation

when this process electrical activation celling and irregular described in the Atria, happens in the ventricles, the arrhythmia is incompatible with life, since the ventricles may not be an effective contraction to pump blood and cardiac arrest occurs in fibrillation, in these cases, not to achieve the cessation of normal electrical activity can be out of unemployment to the patient to achieve this, apply electric current (defibrillation), which produces a total despolarizaci6n of the heart that can later restart activity normal electric.

From the point of view electrocardiographic, ventricular fibrillation is characterized by a total anarchy, where is not possible to recognize any wave, and only contains an irregular tremulation more or less thick line isoelectric with appearance rather than artifacts of an electrocardiogram

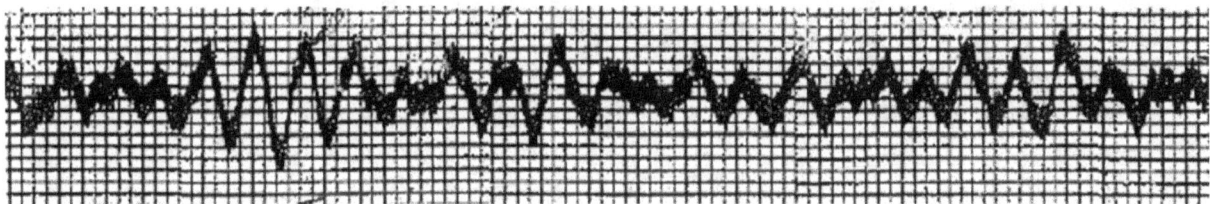

Fig. 3.10 Ventricular fibrillation

Arrhythmias due to alterations in the conduction of the impulse.

Arrhythmias caused by delayed (blockages) are blockages atrioventricular and intraventricular the; the latter by its extent and importance study Chapter 5.

Atrioventricular blockage

Atrioventricular blockages are characterized by a more or less marked difficulty the passage of electrical stimulation through the nodule AV. According to the degree of difficulty, are classified into: first, second and third degrees or complete.

First-degree AV blockage

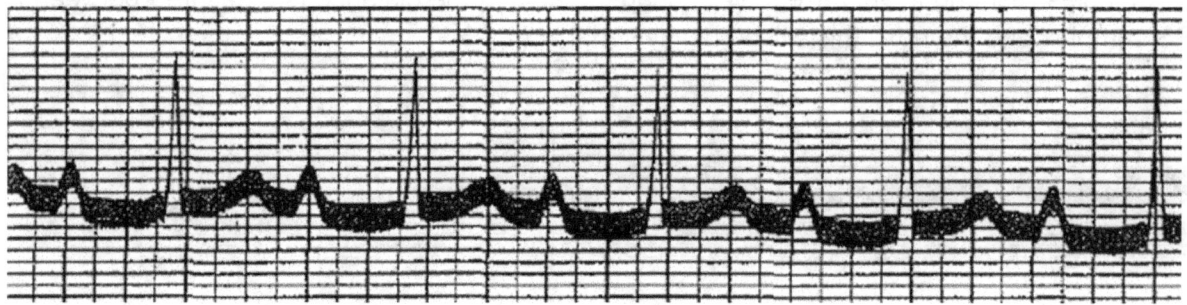

3.11 Blockage AV of first grade with elongation of the PR interval

This type of lock, from the point of view of electrocardiographic, shows that this long PR interval more than usual (0.20 s adult, 0.16 s in the child), but all headphones stimuli are driven, i.e. are followed by their corresponding (fig. 3.11) QRS complex

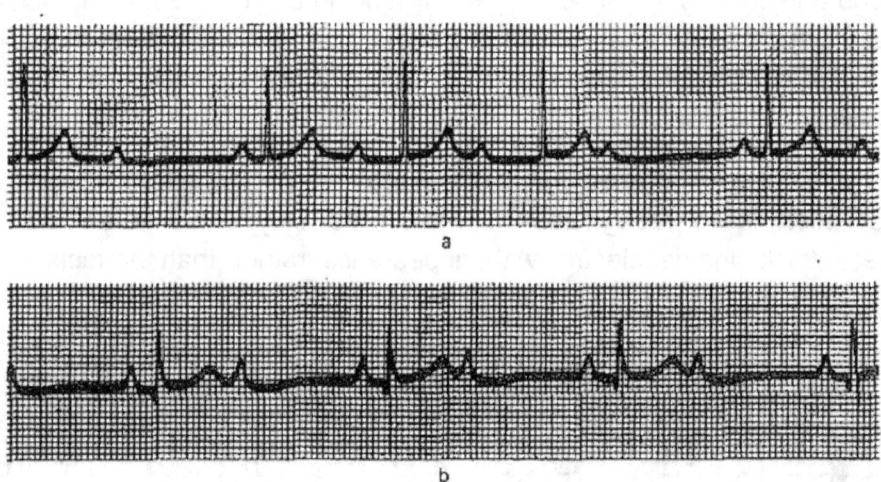

Fig. 3.12 Second degree AV blockade: a, with periods of Wenckebach (the PR is going extending progressively until it appears a P that has no answer); b, Mobitz II with fixed PR type.

Full or third-degree AV blockage

The leading disorder is even more severe, so that no stimulus born in the Atria manages to reach the ventricles; P-waves are produced independently of the QRS complexes. In the path are many more P-waves to QRS complexes, since the ventricles contract with rhythm, always do so at one frequency less than the sinus node.

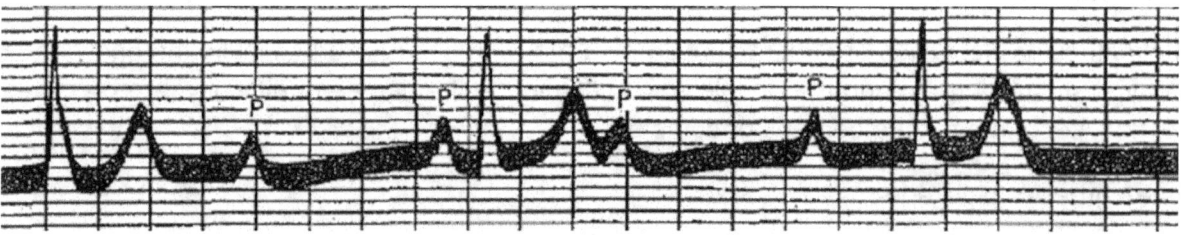

Fig. 3.13 third-degree AV blockage or complete. Note the variability of interval PR and la regularity in a distance RR.

What characterizes this blockade from the electrocardiographic standpoint, is the great variability of the PR interval, which sometimes seems elongated, in other shorts and, occasionally, may appear normal, but this great variability indicates that actually there is no any slur or connection between P waves and QRS complex and both occur independently. Other data of great value is the regularity that exists in time or interval that goes a QRS complex to the next, as the ventricles are beating with own rhythm make it always to a very fixed frequency (fig. (3-13).

Arrhythmias by accelerated

Wolff-Parkinson-White syndrome leading pre-excitation

Stimulation arises as it is usual in the sinus node and activates the Atria which occurs a normal P-wave, but once activated the Atria, passes immediately through an accessory bundle that leads rapidly to the ventricles, which are immediately activated (pre excitation); because of this, appears in the electrocardiogram P-wave and immediately after the QRS complex there is no PR segment; now, the QRS complex presents, in its portion initial apparent disorder which is has been called delta wave, this is because although the stimulus quickly penetrates to the ventricles, does it no ideal way and once in the tentacles began to behave badly. The end of the QRS complex is usually normal appearance, since the stimulus that also penetrates through the AV node ends normally activates the ventricles (fig. 3.14).

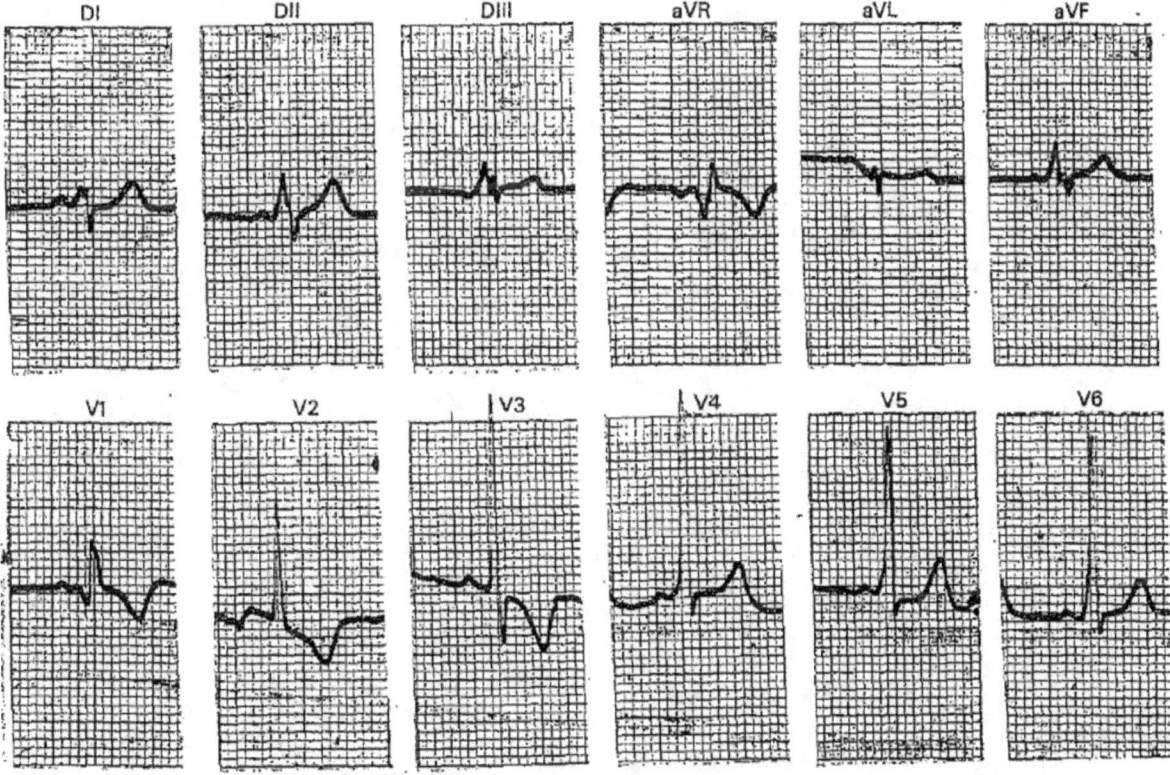

Fig. 3.14 syndrome of Wolff - Parkinson - White. The P wave is immediately followed by the QRS complex widened with initial operating disorders.

The electrocardiographic abnormalities are characterized by the non-existence of the PR segment, the P-wave headquarters immediately before the QRS complex, and this presents deformity in its initial portion motivated by slow interventricular conduction (delta wave).

It should pay special attention to the existence of this syndrome, as alterations that presents the QRS complex may be easily confused with a branch or a ventricular hypertrophy blockage.

Patients with this syndrome are predisposed to suffer from attacks of tachycardia, paroxysmal supra ventricular by a mechanism of reentrant stimulation through the accessory bundle.

4. VENTRICULAR HYPERTROPHY

The ventricular hypertrophy; to increase the thickness of the corresponding muscle mass, determine which increases the magnitude or size of the vector of activation is more space to walk. When the magnitude of this vector is augmented translates into an increase of the voltage of the QRS complex waves

The length or width of the QRS complex against what one might think, is not altered, at least in a remarkable way. The slight widening of QRS that could exist, is not really proportional to the grade of hypertrophy, i.e. does not correspond to the increase of the voltage that presents the QRS complex, it can be inferred that hypertrophies them ventricular increase conduction velocity,

Other alterations that usually produce the ventricular hypertrophy is the inclination of the axis towards the side of the ventricles bloated, since as it is logic, the resulting vector leans toward that side,

Finally the ventricular hypertrophy produced secondary alterations in the wave of recovery or T-wave, which is inverted or flattened those leads that explore the hypertrophied ventricle; the pathophysiology of this reversal of the T wave in the ventricular hypertrophy can be explained by the fact that increasing the thickness of the muscle mass and keep unaltered the coronary supply, causes a degree of relative ischemia of muscle, which is responsible for the alteration of the T-wave to reverse the direction of the vector of recuperate; This will be in more detail in Chapter 6.

To analyze the electrocardiographic abnormalities that produce the ventricular hypertrophy, the following criteria must be present:

- High-voltage QRS complex.
- Deviation of the electric axis
- Reversal or flattening of the T wave, which will analyze each of the types of hypertrophy is studying later.

It is important to warn that not all electrocardiographic criteria must necessarily be present on a path to make the diagnosis of ventricular hypertrophy, but arguably, while larger number of criteria exist the possibility of error will be smaller. As same, before tackling the alterations the hypertrophy electrocardiographic is advisable to review with regard to high voltage electrical axis of the QRS complex.

LEFT VENTRICULAR HYPERTROPHY

High-voltage QRS complex. The V6 R wave is more than 25 mm, or presents an index of Sokolow (wave V6 R more the VI S wave) with more than 35 mm; V2 S-waves with less than 25 mm, and the R-wave of aVL has more than 13 mm.

Electric axis deviation. The electric shaft is diverted into left and produces predominantly positive QRS patterns in DI and DIII negatives.

Disturbances in the wave of recuperate. (T-wave). The waves are flattened or inverted on the left precordial VS and V6 and 01 and aVL, discordant with the main encouragement of the QRS complex.

It is good to warn now that the diagnosis of certainty of the ventricular hypertrophy, as well as the branch blockades, they must always be confirmed in precordial leads since the anatomical position of the heart is able to change orientation of the vectors in the derivations of the members.

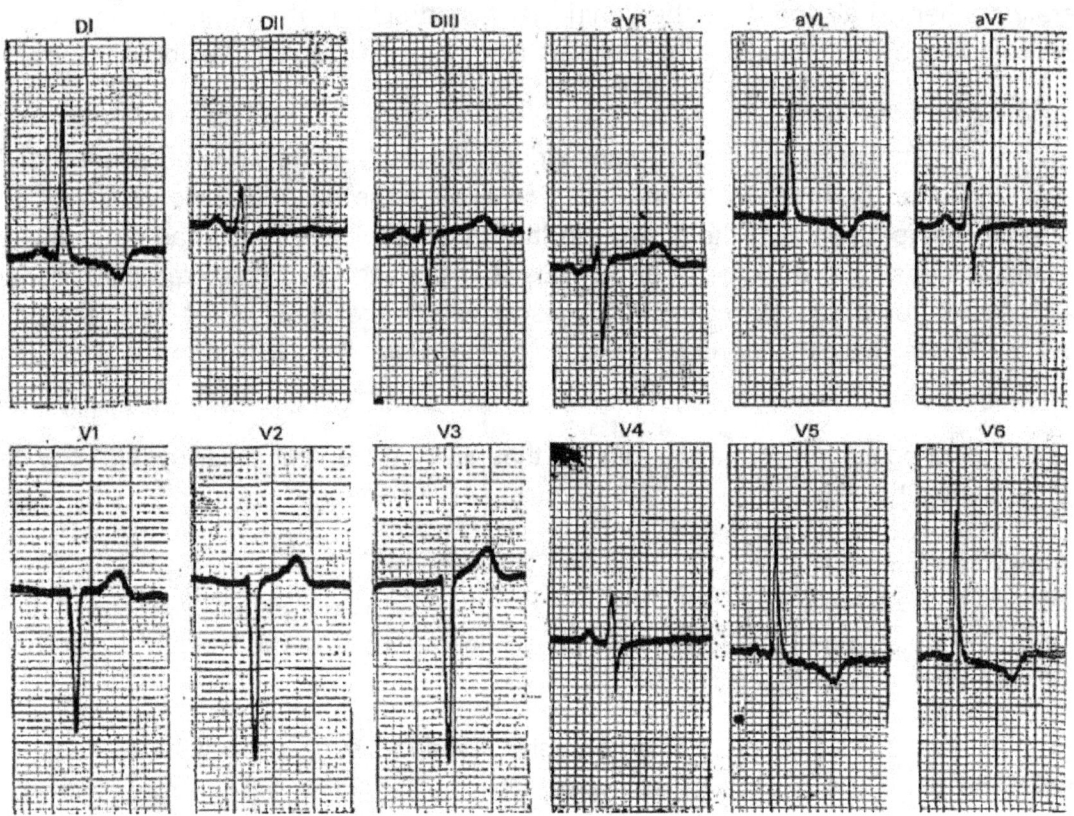

Fig. 4.1. Left ventricular hypertrophy: a, with electrical axis deviated towards the left: b, with electrical axis in normal position.

For instance, when the heart has a rotating around its longitudinal axis that determines the left ventricle is aimed down, resting on the diaphragm, the vectors of activation of the left, rather than move towards the left ventricle, projected downward, and appear high voltages of the QRS leads complex lower (DII, DIII aVF), as to the aVL derivation It is located upward and to the left, exhibits a QRS pattern with a strong predominance of negative, as if it were a right ventricular hypertrophy, when in reality it's a left ventricular hypertrophy in a heart electric upright. The (only way to not make a mistake, is the confirmation of the diagnosis in the precordial leads (fig. 4.2).

Given the above, it is advisable to bear in mind that the left ventricular hypertrophy not necessarily has to turn the shaft to the left, but that can occur in the presence of a normal electric shaft or even in a vertical position, which can occasionally lead to confusion with the derivations of the members in right ventricular hypertrophy.

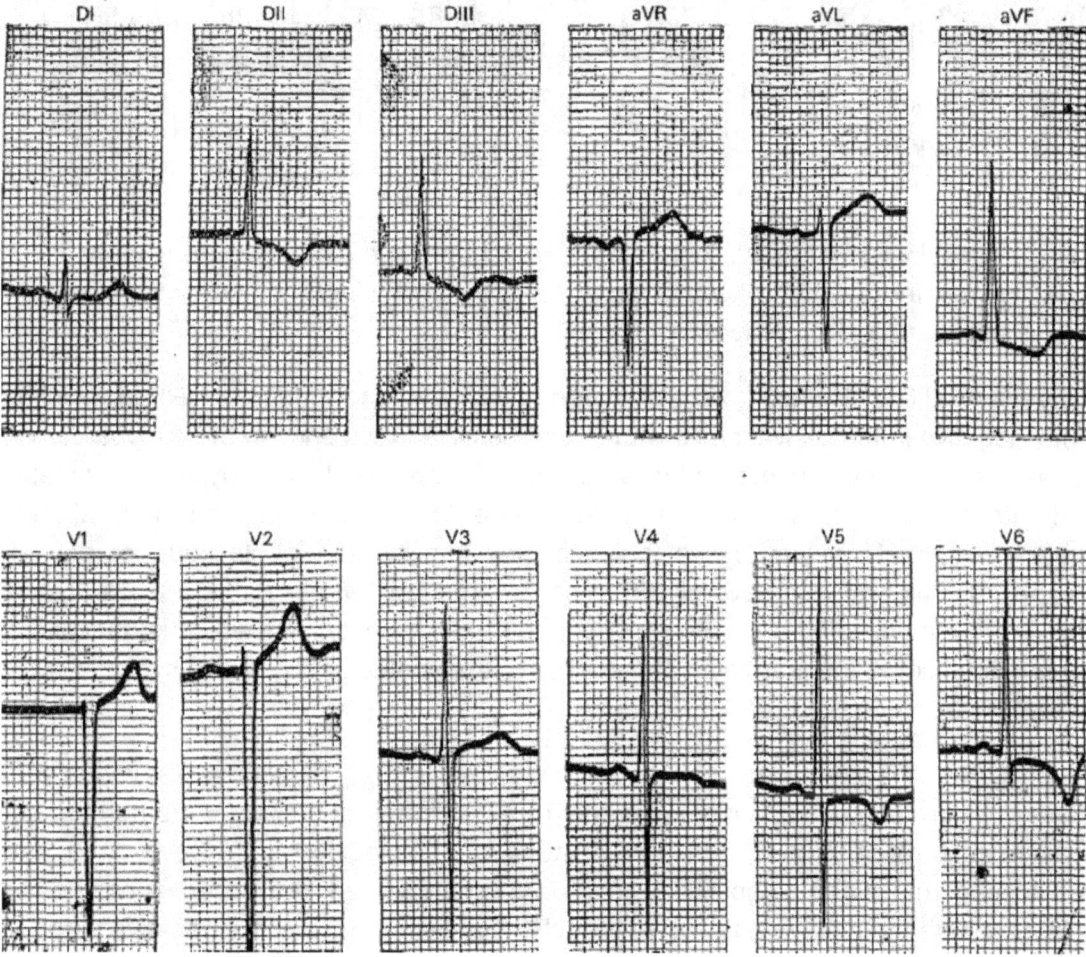

Fig. 4.2. Left ventricular hypertrophy. Index of Sokolow extremely altered with strong investment of waves Ten V5 and V6. Electrical axis in a normal position; Electric upright, left ventricular heart projected their potential down (DII, DIII and VF). Note that in this case the shunt to VL is predominantly negative and simulates a right ventricular hypertrophy that does not exist.

RIGHT VENTRICULAR HYPERTROPHY

High-voltage QRS complex. V1 R wave is more than 10 mm, and although it does not reach this far, predominates over the S wave; i.e., relationship r/s greater than 1. If this wave R is a disorder of driving in their ascending Ramus (indenting or filling) it still has more value. A wave S

VL is presented with a depth greater than 10 mm and there is predominance of Ia positive wave in the QRS complex of a VR.

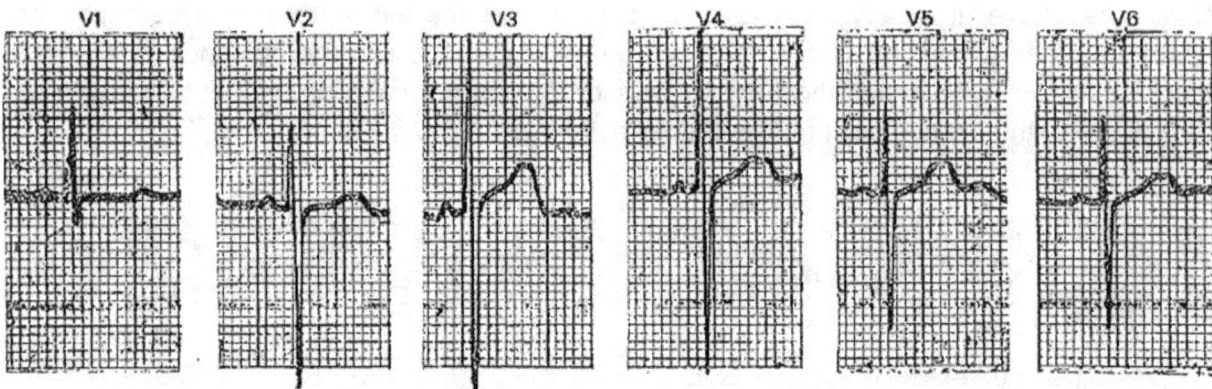

Fig. 4.3. Right ventricular hypertrophy. Right axis deviation, prevalence of R in derivation to VR, strong negativity in referral to VL R wave predominantly in the right precordial leads, with conduction disturbances began. T waves are normal.

Electric axis deviation. The electrical axis is deviated to the right, and produces QRS complexes predominantly negative in the derivation DI with strong positive prevalence in the derivation DIII. To the difference left ventricular hypertrophy, is rare to find a right ventricular hypertrophy that is not diverted into the right axis, and the most severe lead it upward and right already (indeterminate position); However, occasionally, if they coexist with a blockage of the left anterior fascicle, the shaft may be severely deviated towards the; left since this disease, as we will see later, is characterized by producing a strong left axis deviation. Anyway, just that in the hypertrophy left ventricular, the diagnosis of certainty of the ventricular hypertrophy Right must be corroborated in the precordial leads.

The disorders recovery (T-wave) wave. Right ventricular hypertrophy can cause the investment of waves have the right precordial leads. A T-wave invested in the derivation V1 is normal, but when it goes more beyond. V2, V3, etc., in an adult is pathological, and above all, in the presence of an abnormal QRS complex. T waves are also inverted in the derivations of the members disagree with the main orientation of the QRS complex; i.e., become negative in those ramifications that have complex QRS with strong positive prevalence and the reverse.

HYPERTROPHY VENTRICULAR COMBINED

Suspected ventricular or combined ventricular hypertrophy in the following situations:

1. When there are bypass V1 criteria of high voltage to make the diagnosis of right ventricular hypertrophy to bypass V6 existence criteria for diagnosis of left ventricular hypertrophy in AI. 2. when there are patterns isodiphasic of high voltage (R and S of more than 20 mm waves) on the precordial VI to V 4 accompanying patterns isodiphasic of high voltage (R and S of more than 10 mm) in two or more of the derivations of the members.

Usually there is no marked axial deviation and the disorder in the vein of recuperate (T-wave) may or not be present. Is good warn that the criteria of high voltage of the complex QRS in the child, as well as the deviation axial, can vary based on the age (should review the chapter 7).

Finally, it is accepted there are overloads of volume, which produce more expansion and an increase in the thickness of the ventricular wall; These overloads of volume or diastolic, mean which for the right ventricle in the existence of polyphase patterns or double R in the right precordial leads, with high voltage, and for the left ventricle on the existence in the more deep Q waves left precordial 3 mm with very high and symmetrical in the V6 deviation T waves.

The pathophysiology of these disorders is still not well clarified.

VENTRICULAR OVERLOAD TYPES

The concepts of overloading diastolic and systolic were introduced in electrocardiography by Dr. Enrique Cabrera and collaborators.

The ventricles in each contraction driven out a certain amount of blood, which must overcome some resistance. The type of overload is determined both by the resistance that must be overcome the ventricles to eject blood, like pair volume which must expel in each contraction.

Systolic overload

occurs when there is difficulty to expel the blood due to increased resistance, which must beat the ventricle (post load); as consequence of this ventricle increases the thickness of its walls, therefore, systolic overload is recognized in the path by alterations that denote the thickness of the muscle mass increase and the consequent deficits of oxygen (relative ischemia) since the coronary contribution is the same regardless of the grade of muscle hypertrophy. Therefore appear QRS patterns with strong positive prevalence and T waves flattened or inverted about the ramifications that explore the affected ventricle: precordial (V1 or V2) for the right ventricle (fig. 4.4) and left precordial leads (V5 or V6) for the left ventricle (fig. 4.4 b).

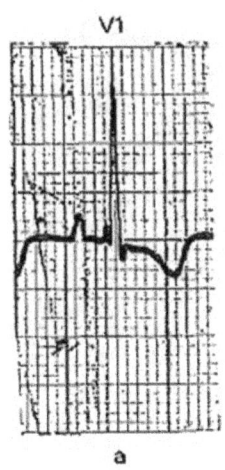
a

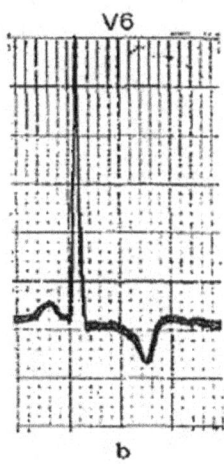
b

Fig. 4.4 Systolic overloading: a, right ventricular and b, left ventricular diastolic overload

in this case overload is caused by the increased inflow of blood into the ventricles (preload); as a result the affected ventricle dilates rather than exaggerating it. The pathophysiology of the electrocardiographic abnormalities that appear in the diasto1icas overloads has not been universally accepted; These alterations consist of the appearance of polyphase type QRS patterns or double R on the right precordial (VI or V2) diastolic right ventricular (fig. 4.5A) overloads while diastolic left ventricular overload leads to the appearance in the left precordial leads (V5 or V6) of QRS complexes with something deeper than normal Q waves (more than 3 mm) , together with the presence of very high and symmetrical T waves (fig. 4.5 b).

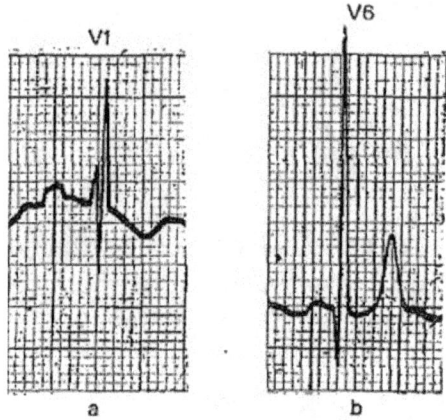

Fig. 4.5 Diastolic Overload: a, right ventricular: b, left ventricular

5. INTRA VENTRICULAR BLOCKAGES

In Chapter 5 explained the nodule atrioventricular continuous downward with the bundle of His, which after a short ride is divided into two main branches, right and left, which are distributed by the appropriate ventricle.

The right branch of the get of His, is long, thin and cylindrical, and remains indivisible until their networks are done at the level of the muscle papillary previous of the ventricle right. The left branch of the bundle of His, after a short ride, is divided into two issues, one earlier and other posterior, which are distributed in the anterior and posterior portions of the left ventricle, at the level of the papillary muscles. These two issues, the former is the longer and more vulnerable, while the back is short, thick and generally crashes less frequently.

BRANCH BLOCKAGES. GENERAL CHARACTERISTICS

The term bundle branch block is used to designate a functional or organic disorder that slows down or disrupts the conduction of the wave of activation at the level of one of the branches of the bundle of HIS.

As it has been seen in the normal activation of the ventricles, the activation wave penetrates simultaneously by both branches of the bundle of His, right and left, and the ventricular portion to the interventricular septum in the middle region, is the first to be activated via the left branch bundle; now, once activated the septum, the stimulus begins to simultaneously activate both ventricles, and the vector 2 ventricular activation is, as it has been seen, a resulting vector of the activation of both ventricles.

Obstructed or impaired handling by one of the branches, electrical stimulation is distributed by branch unscathed, to activate, in the first place, the ventricle which has blocked branch, and later wave of activation directed from the ventricle which has been activated to one who has blocked branch, to activate it; This makes the ventricular activation, which is usually done in a simultaneous way, if there a bundle branch block, is made in an asynchronous way, i.e. first activates the ventricle which has the branch free and secondly the ventricle which has blocked branch; This brings as a consequence, in the first place. A delay in the time of ventricular activation, which dramatically increases the width or length of the complex QRS.

Secondly, the fact that stimulation to activate the ventricle which has blocked branch, has to be distributed or follow a path, which is not ideal for driving, should be assessed which brings as a consequence that in addition to being wide, QRS complex present what we call "conduction disturbances", that they mean the layout by the fact that the QRS complex loses the thin and crisp stroke that is characteristic, and presents: thickening or smearing, dents and irregularities of its waves.

Thirdly, branch locks usually give rise to disorders in the wave of recovery (T-wave), which is reversed; This investment is due to the fact that to extend the time of ventricular activation, the cells of the layer sub endocardial can recover or begin the recovery process, which therefore invests its sense advancing endocardial or epicardial, which determines, at the same time, the reversal of the direction of the vector of recovery.

Finally, it is important to know that to establish the diagnosis of bundle branch block, is essential requirement having a sinus rhythm ECG and PR interval is normal; This indicates that stimulation was normally born in the sinus node, the Atria were activated normally, stimulation through the AV node and the bundle of His (PR segment), and entering only from here on, i.e. when the stimulus by the branches, is that the disorder starts driving; with this false locks of branch, as the syndrome of Wolff-Parkinson-White, in which there is no segment PR, in addition to discard the extrasystole and ventricular rhythms, in which deformed QRS complex is not preceded by the P wave is discarded.

In short, the electrocardiographic criteria for the diagnosis of bundle branch block are:

- The presence of sinus with link to V (PR) rhythm normal.
- Widened QRS complexes (more than 0.10 s adult and 0.08 in the child).
- QRS complex with conduction disorder.
- Disorders in the wave recuperate T (inverted T waves)

To then explain what are the characteristics of the layout, if the block is right bundle branch or left bundle branch."

Right bundle branch block.

In the right bundle branch block, the stimulus enters from the left branch and produces the first activation of the septum (vector 1) vector (fig. 5.1 to); is subsequently activated the region of the tip of the heart and the left ventricular wall, which leads to the emergence of a second resulting vector of these triggers, which has a very similar to the vector resultant 2 normal activation (fig. 5.1 b); i.e., the beginning of the complex QRS has few changes in right bundle branch block; then however, there is a third vector late directed from left to right, caused by the wave of activation which passes from the left ventricle to the right, vector ventricle which is very delayed in its progress, is heading wide a route that is not AI suitable for driving (fig. 5.1c). This third vector causes the appearance of a wide S wave and conduction disturbances in the ramifications that explore the heart from the left side (VS, V6 and DI); While the right branch (DI and aVR), produced a second wave wide R and with conduction disturbances, resulting in the classic pattern in double R (fig. 5.1).

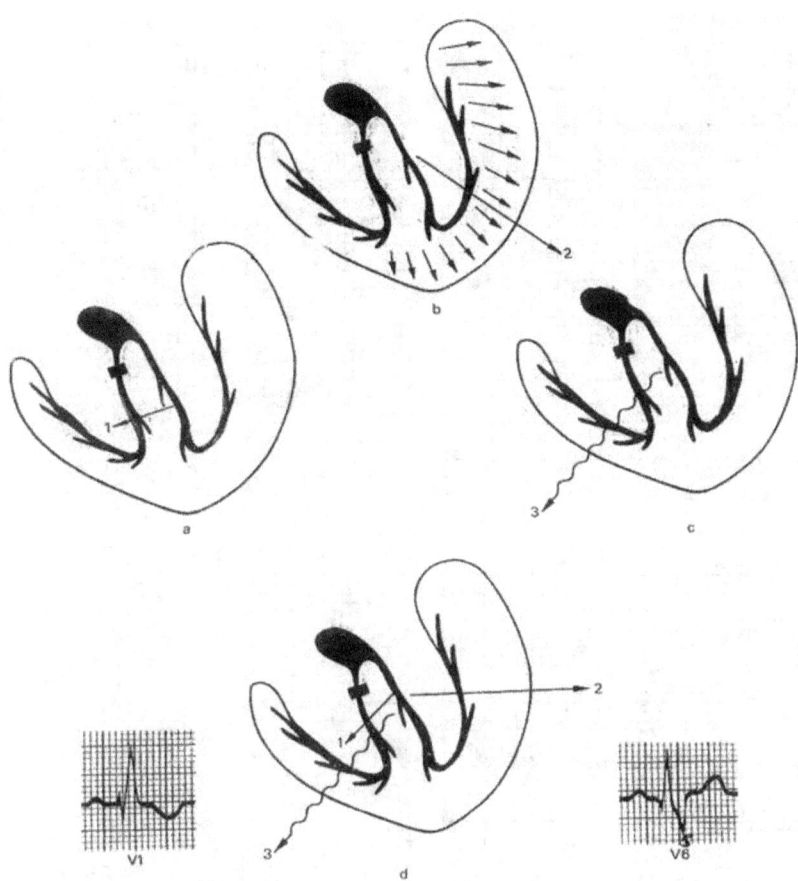

Fig 5.1 Right branch blockage

Generally, blockage of the right branch bundle is recognized easily in the right precordial, to produce the pattern in RR, first by the activation of the septum and the second wide and impaired driving as a result of the abnormal activation of the right ventricle. As the blockade becomes full, the first R-wave tends to disappear (fig. 5.2)

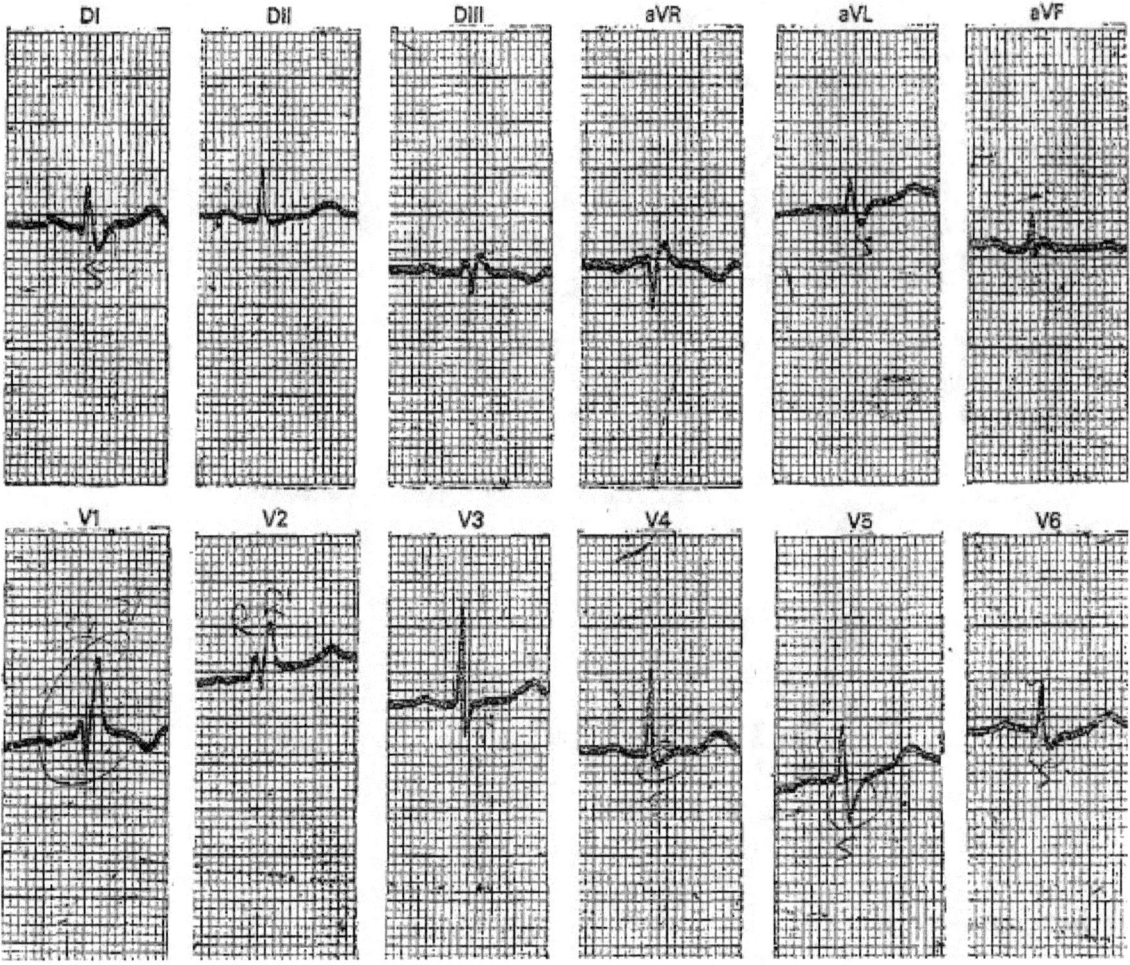

Fig. 5.2 right bundle branch block. Observe double R in the right precordial leads, and the wide S wave and pattern with the disorder operating on the left leads Dl, aVL, V5 and V6.

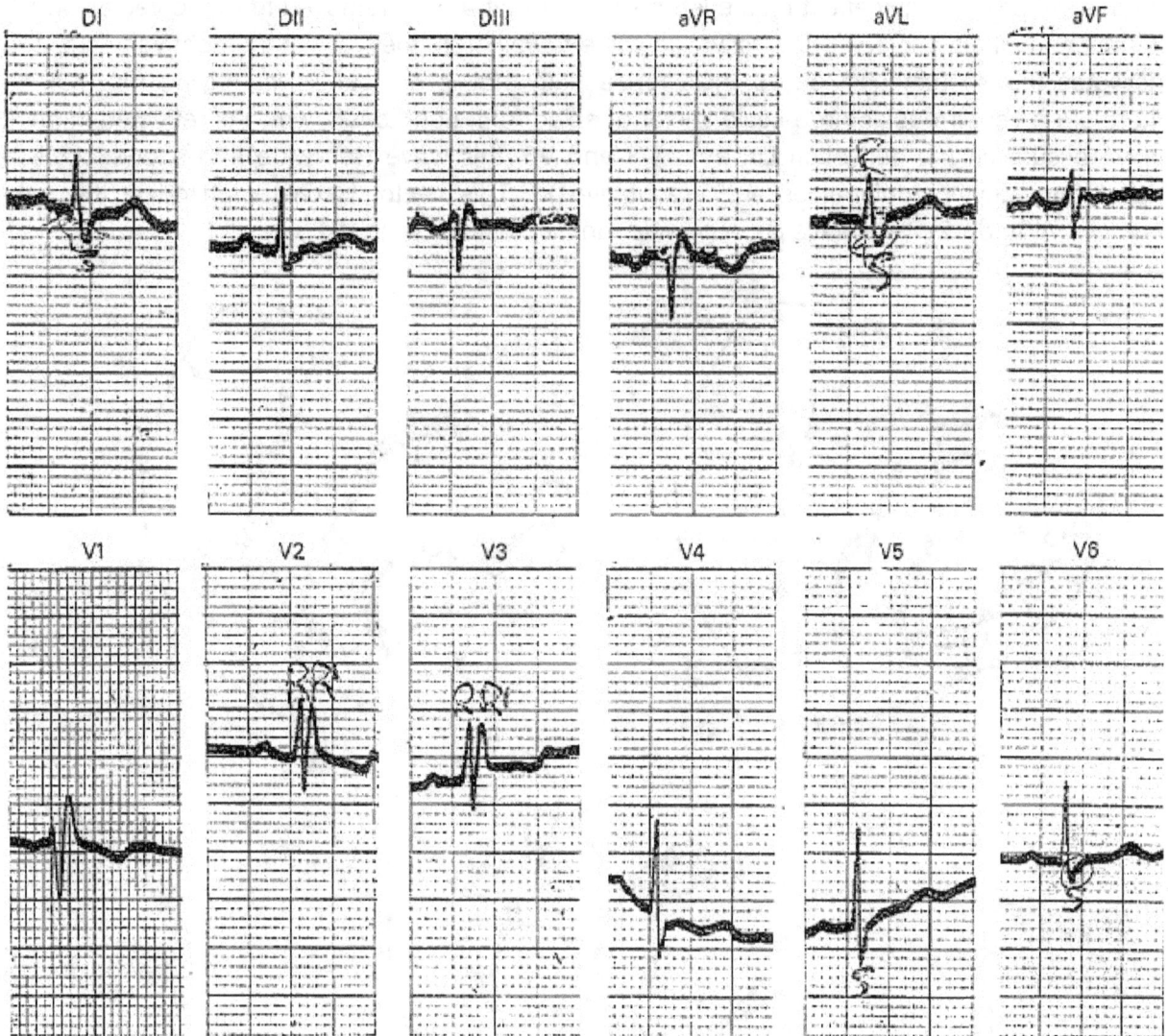

Fig 5.3 Right branch blockage. Observe the QRS interval widened with double R in the right precordial pattern as well as filling of the ascending ramus of the S wave on the left leads DI, aVL, V5 and V6.

In the left bundle branch blockage left bundle branch block, alteration in the ventricular activation is much more marked than in right bundle branch block; interventricular septum is not activated in the first instance, as is well known its activation occurs via the left branch bundle; as a result, the absence of Q waves on the DI, aVL left leads V5 and V6.

This blockage is activated first is in the right ventricular, which produces vector activation directed

1 from left to right (fig. 5.4 to), at the same time, this vector that displays a small R wave in a derivation that is registering the potential from the right side, as for example, V 1, but

It does not produce any effect on the left deviations that are far removed from the vector, which is rather small magnitude. Then activation wave travels from the walls of the right ventricle, and activates the septum and left ventricle, on a path that is not suited for driving (fig. 5.4 b); therefore a very irregular large-scale vector directed from right to left, which is reflected in an R wave occurs (in the derivation DI, aVL, VS and V6, this wave Res wide and shows obvious upset from driving (deformities and irregularities). This vector is characterized in the right branch (V1 and V2), by a wave S deep, wide, and impaired driving (fig 5.4c)

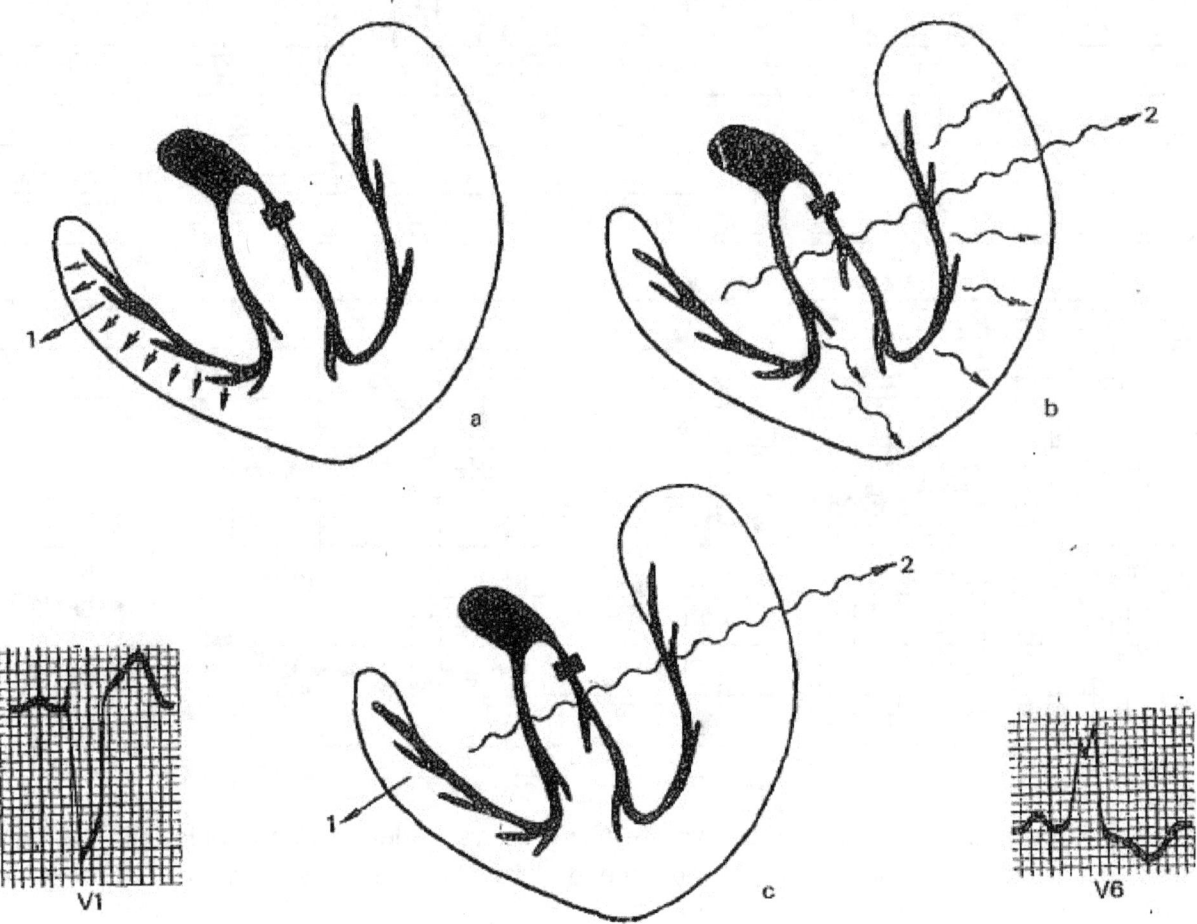

Fig 5.4 for your interest left bundle branch block, is presented in Figure 5.5 a blocking of left bundle branch with all features alterations, while missing the investment recovery wave or wave T (atypical left bundle branch block) in Figure 5.6.

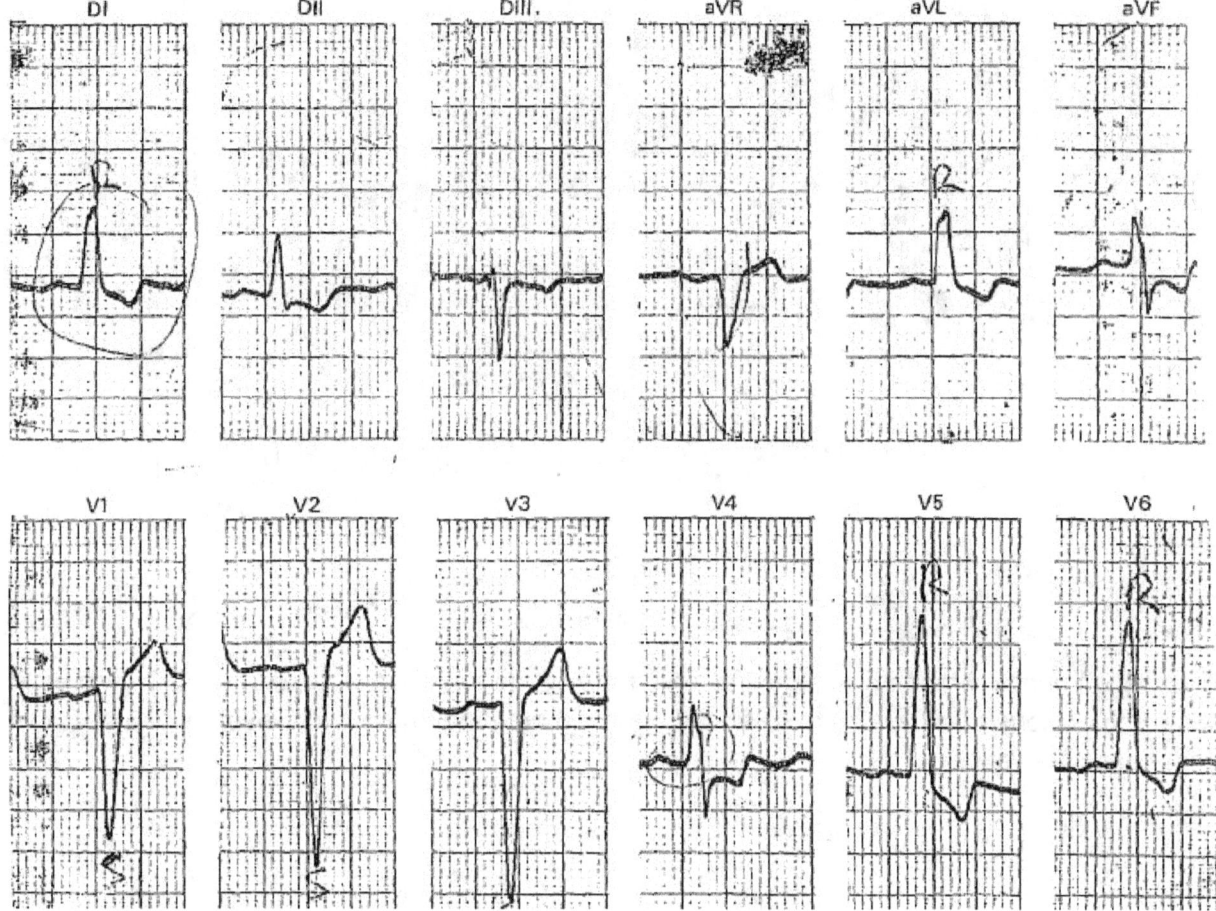

Fig. 5.5 left bundle branch blockage. Observe the widening of the QRS complex and the unique R waves with disorders of operating on the left leads DI, aVL. V5 and V6, as well as inverted T waves.

It is good to repeat here, that the diagnosis or certainty of branch as well as the of the hypertrophy locks must be in the precordial to avoid errors, modifications that the changes in position of the heart can give to the path in the derivations of the members; in this regard, remember that DI and aVL are leads the left-oriented and normally they should scan the wall of the left ventricle, except for those cases in which the heart by virtue of its rotation around the longitudinal axis, projects the ventricle down making it rest on the diaphragm, in such cases, patterns of the left ventricle they transmit to the inferior leads (DII DIII and aVF)

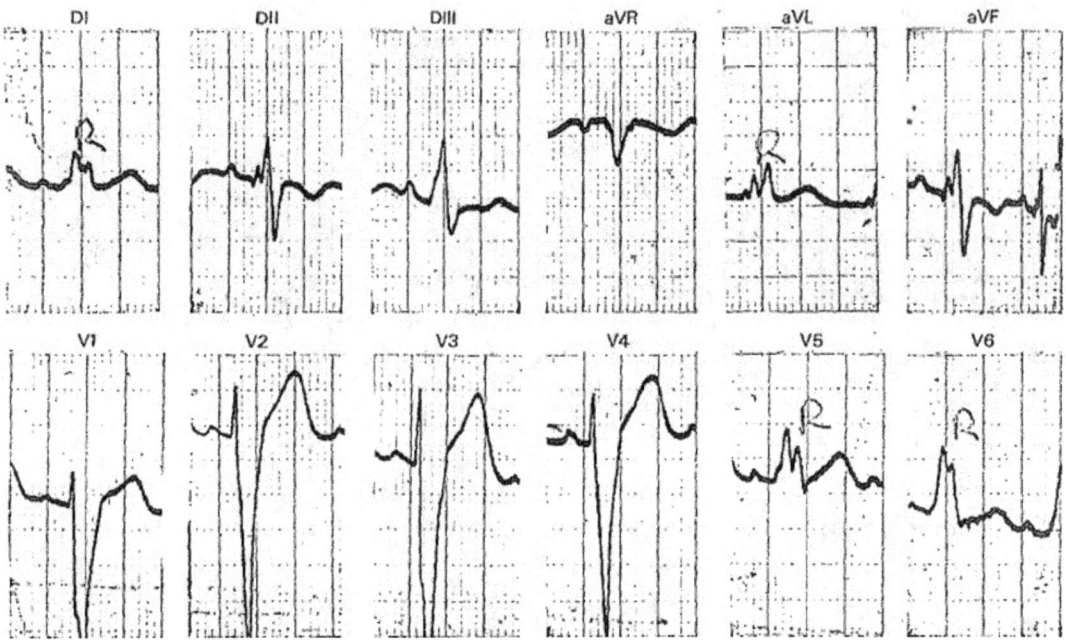

Fig. 5.6 left bundle branch blockage. Observe marked increase in the duration of QRS waves R wide with obvious disorders on the left leads. Please note that there is no reversal of the waves keep these derivations.

Fascicular blocks

The Foundation of the fascicular blocks lies in the conception that the stimulus that it descends the left branch bundle to activate the left ventricle, follows the two divisions of this beam, the previous and the later, nearly simultaneously body by activating the corresponding walls of the left ventricle, which shows that block is one of the subdivisions, there is a delay of 0.02 s or something more in the entire area of the wall of the left ventricle where the booklet is distributed.

Left anterior fascicular block

If the anterior fascicle is blocked, the stimulus is driven by the further subdivision, which It points to the diaphragm, and first active portions of the left ventricle and then inferior posterior, the face anterosuperior; CS logical that the final activation of the QRS complex forces move away from the expensive diaphragmatic and pointing up, diverting the electric of the QRS complex markedly basin left.

Slow activation and the upper front of the left ventricle regions late, leads to a delay in the activation bypass which studies the upper part of the left ventricle (aVL), not so in V6, which studies the part low of the ventricle. The point of view electrocardiographically, this type of blockage from fascicular is characterized by:

1. in standard derivations there are strong left axis deviation, with QRS complexes with positive prevalence in DI and predominantly negative in DII and DIII. 2 delay in time of registration in the aVL, the derivation which shows a somewhat enlarged and light filling R wave, while the R wave

of the derivation V6 is narrow and does conduction disturbances; This is due to the asynchronism in the activation between high portions (aVL) and low (V6) of the left ventricle. The total duration of the QRS (width) not this altered (fig. 5.7) complex.

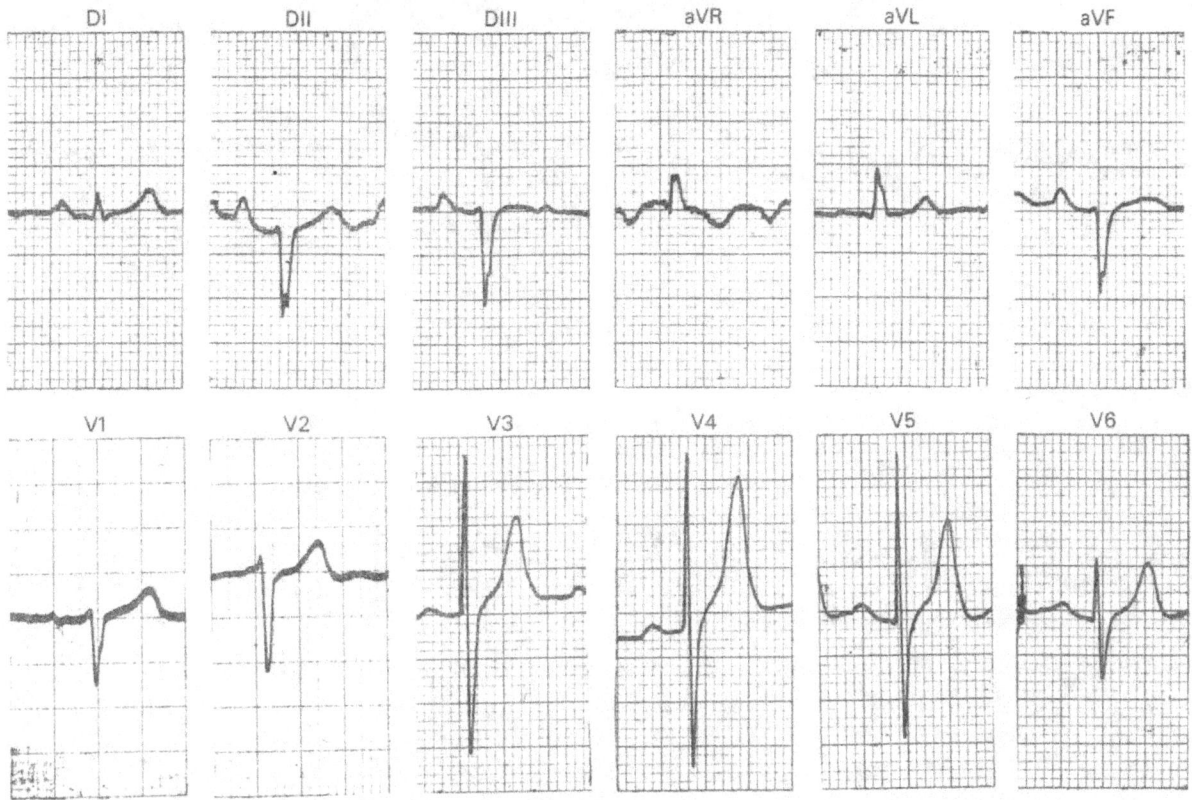

Fig. 5.7 left anterior fascicular block. Note the strong left axis deviation. The R-wave of longer duration than V6 the aVL. Despite the strong left axis deviation, there is no criteria of high voltage, or alterations in wave T to make the diagnosis of left ventricular hypertrophy.

Blockage left anterior fascicular with right bundle branch blockage

This association is not uncommon. From the point of view electrocardiographic, bi-fascicular block is characterized because the layout maintains the criteria already set forth in the left anterior fascicular block, Diagnostics and the concomitant right bundle branch block is diagnosed in right precordial leads where it appears a pattern polyphasic or double R, or an R wave broadband with apparent disorder of terminal driving. On the left leads DI and V6, appears also the S wave broadband and with disorders of operating features of the right block (fig. 5.8).

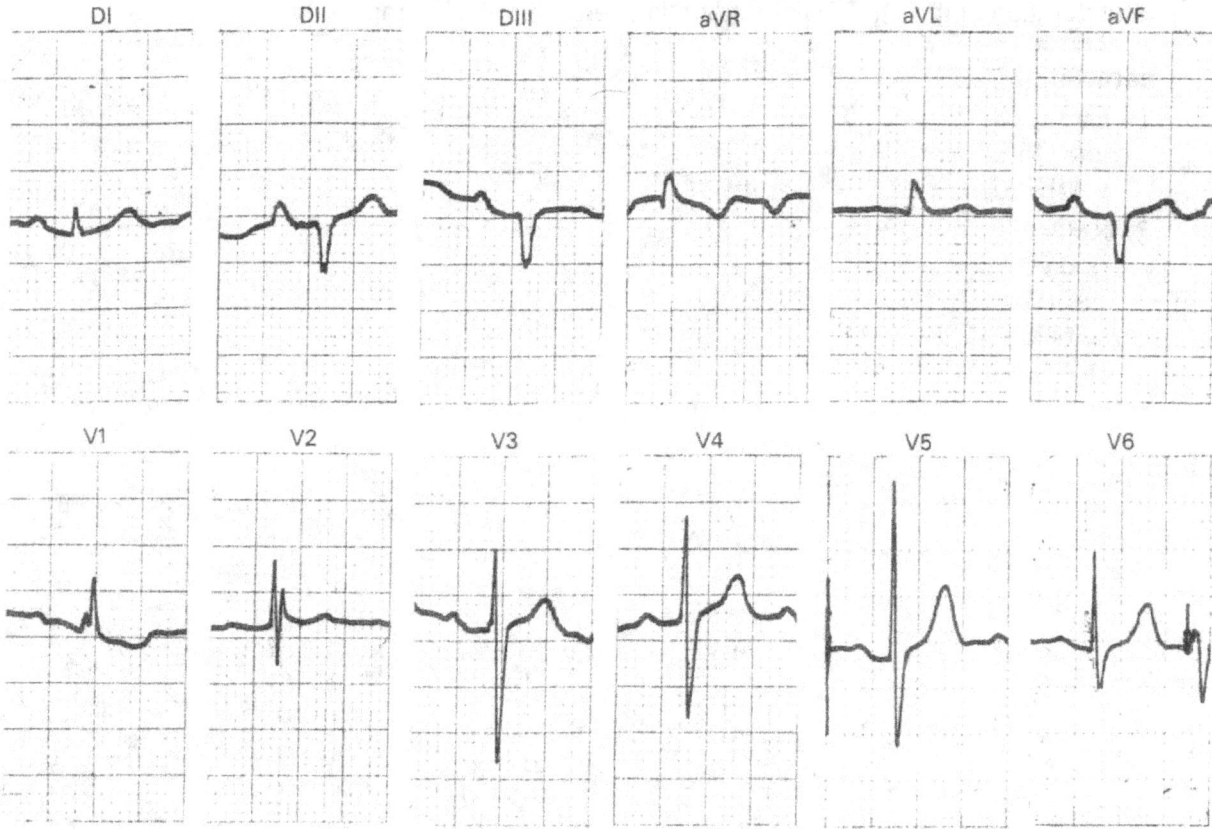

Fig. 5.8 blockage left anterior fascicular with right bundle branch block. Strong deviation of the axis to the left, as well as different in the R in aVL and V6 wave width identify the blockage of the left anterior fascicle. The R-wave broadband and with disorders of operating in the right precordial in the same way as wide S-waves and smears on the left leads V5 and V6 identified the right bundle branch block.

Left posterior fascicular block isolated from the left rear fascicle, blocking is not frequent, as this issue less vulnerable area of intraventricular conduction. In these cases, the stimulus is driven by the previous branch and they appear as more early forces of left ventricular activation, those oriented upwards and forwards; the left ventricle posteroinferior portion is activated late. Thus explained shaft electric store upright positions, as well as delay in activation, observed in the derivations DII, DIII, aVF, and occasionally in V6.

From the electrocardiographic point of view, this lock is characterized by: leads estimate there are right axis deviation, with predominant S bypass-waves

DI and patterns are predominantly positive type QR DII and DIII leads; R waves of these derivations, tend to show changes in the driving.

2. The time activation leads aVF and V6, studying also the posteroinferior portions of the left ventricle, this retarded alga; however, the total length or width of the QRS complex remains unchanged

6. CORONARY INSUFFICIENCY

Alteration that occurs when blood supply to the myocardia through the arteries called coronary insufficiency coronary arteries is not adequate. The degree of this deficit can range from chronic forms to the more acute.

CARDIOPHATIC ISQUEMIC

Ischemic Heart disease occurs when a disruption of the contribution of blood to the par myocardia obstruction of coronary flow, myocardial irrigation deficit translates into a series of electrocardiographic, mainly at the level of the ST segment and t wave abnormalities

The severity of myocardial, so alterations as electrocardiographic are conditioned by the greater or lesser changes degree of deficit; so, for example, if what is happening is only a decrease of watering I blood pair a partial obstruction of the vasa or affected vessels, presents a process called ischemia. But if the occlusion of the vessel is full, this phase of ischemia established sharply determined quickly a degree of deterioration of the myocardial cells much more severe, Hamada lesion, and finally more the part injured cells were necrotic.

Classification

From the tip of life practical heart disease ischemic can be classified into two groups:

1. when there is only a reduction in irrigation blood "ischemia", angor pectoris, or angina pectoris, which from the point of view of electrocardiographic manifests itself usually (not always) by the so-called signs of myocardial ischemia, and whose clinical picture can be very variable, especially , what the painful manifestations are concerned.
2. When the contribution blood ceases altogether in certain area of the myocardia, and infarction of the myocardia, in which, accompanying severe ischemia, are stages more serious deterioration as injury and finally is the necrosis.

Signs electrocardiographic

The stadiums heart disease ischemic described above translates in the electrocardiogram as shown in Figure 6.1, and are described below:

1. Ischemia is recognized pair T-wave inversion

2. In the lesion occurs a drop of ST-segment.

3. Necrosis translates into the presence of waves Q features abnormal, called Q waves pathological (infarction).

Pathophysiology

Below explains, roughly described electrocardiographic changes physiopathology. Ischemia leads to the inversion of T wave because when is present on the surface exterior of the myocardia, alteration produced in these cells of the layer surface, it makes to the recovery vector (T-wave) start in the cells of the layers deeper and to reverse pair both its sense, propagandized inside out.

The lesion presents drop of ST-segment (more than 1 mm), because it causes a partial depolarization in the injured area, appears an abnormal electric current called current of injury, which is in charge of the unevenness of this segment. In the presence of Q wave necrosis pathological is the necrotic tissue is electrically dead, so is other and does not bring any vector to power electrical balance during ventricular activation; then, dominate the vectors that are in the area opposite to necrosis, bringing as they deviate from the electrode that is exploring the area of necrosis, as a result that enroll a large initial negative wave in the QRS complex.

Whatever Q waves usually are present in normal electrocardiograms, is necessary to point out the diagnostic criteria to identify a pathological Q-wave (Q); Indeed, the normal Q-wave, as we know, is caused by the activation of the interventricular septum and is a negative wave initial small, that rarely happens 2-3 mm deep, also is narrow and only appears in the ramifications that explore the left ventricle V4, V6, DI, VS and aVL (if the heart is in a vertical position, LHC appear in DII) (, DIII and aVF, but always with the characteristics already mentioned).

Criteria Q-wave pathological diagnostics

1. Depth. It is much more profound that a normal Q, especially when compared with the R wave. A Q-wave that is greater than 25% of the R-wave, is pathological.
2. Length. The pathological Q-wave is wider than usual, usually greater than 0.03 s duration.
3. Can show (nicks, smears) conduction disturbances.

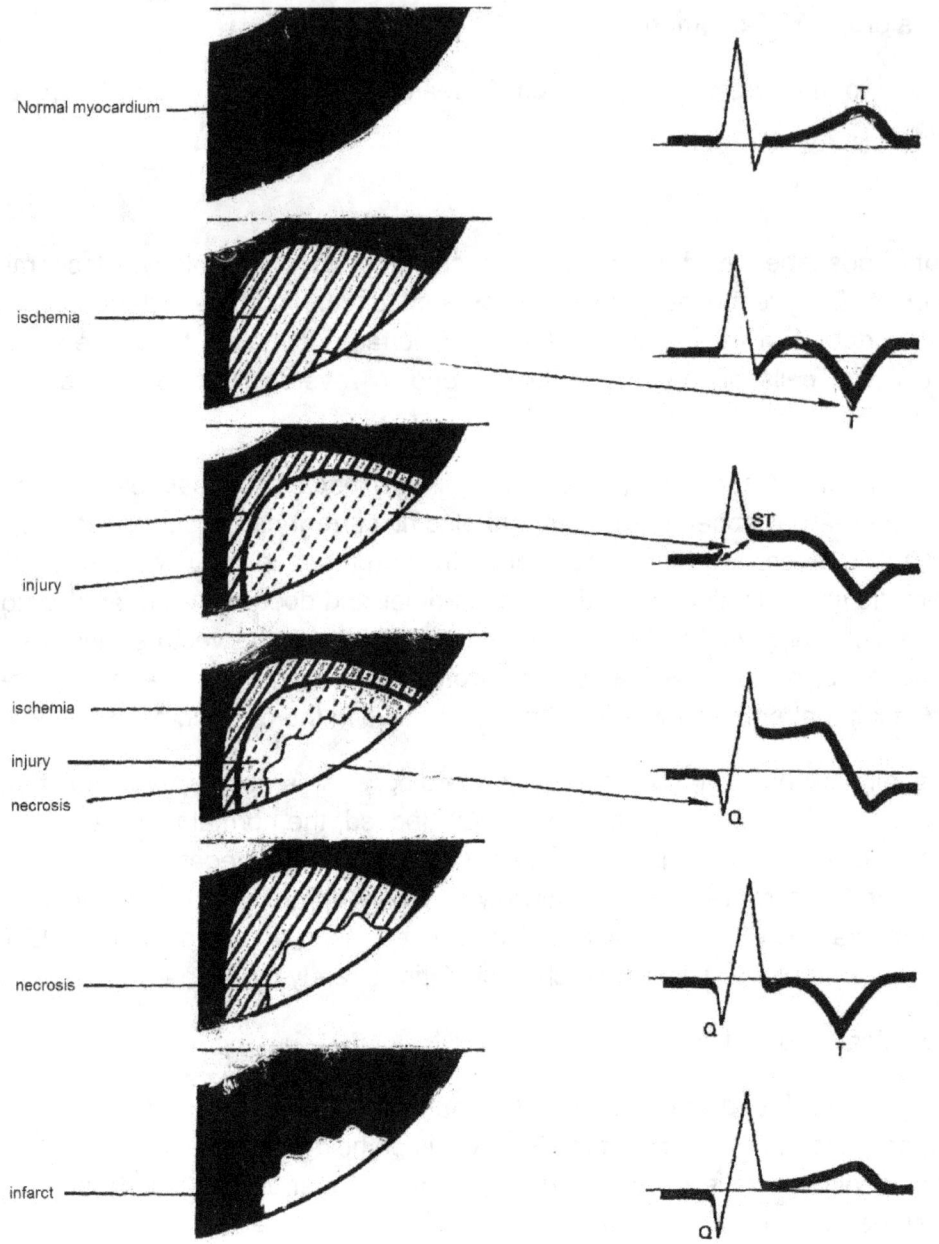

Fig 6.1 Evolutionary States of infarction.

It is convenient to know that there are situations that may give rise to the emergence of large Q waves in some of the electrocardiogram leads, unless it's a heart attack; so for example: in cases of left ventricular hypertrophy or left bundle branch block may appear big QS in the precordial deviations standing waves, even up to V4, which are not due to necrosis, but are easily discarded, since in these cases the large waves QS are positive accompanied by T waves.

Similarly, the shunt DIII may appear occasionally a Q-wave very deep because of the position of the heart. Minus you value if not appear together this large DII and aVF leads Q-wave, or if this

Q-wave is modified when taking the bypass DIII asking the patient that makes an inspiration deep to vary the position of the heart.

MYOCARDIAL INFARCTION

Positive diagnosis

The positive diagnosis is performed to identify the signs of heart attack; in the electrocardiogram these are:

- Pathological Q wave (necrosis)
- Positive slope of the (injury) ST-segment
- Inverted T wave (ischemia) (fig. 6-1).

The mentioned changes that constitute the so-called signs of infarction occur when the infarcted area opens to the surface gap of the heart (most of the time), but occasionally the infarcted area can be opened toward the inside of the ventricle (towards the endocardium), in which case in the solo path appears as alteration a strong slope ST-segment with a very positive T wave negative (fig. 6.2 to). Rarely also the infarcted area does not open to external or internal surface, but it remains in the thickness of the muscle (infarction intramural) and in this case the (single alteration is the presence of a strongly-inverted T wave and symmetrical (fig. 6.2 b).) In the diagnosis of these heart attacks are the manifestations of great value patient clinics, as well as the determination of enzymes.

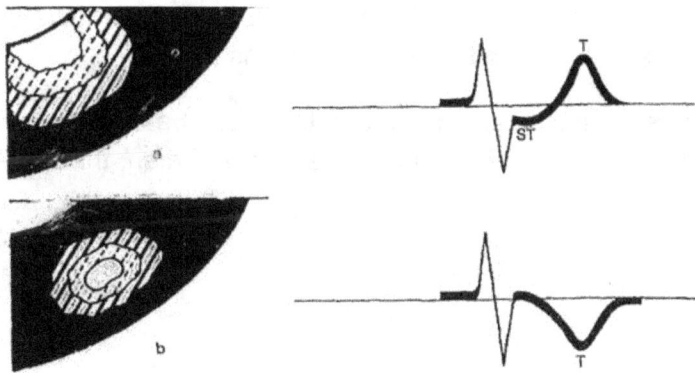

Fig 6.2 infarction: a. sub-endocardial: b. intramural. Both with the corresponding electrocardiographic abnormalities.

Diagnostics evolutionary

In houses of survival of the patient, the infarction passes through three stages:

1. Acute stage, is characterized by a frank predominance of the lesion, i.e. the marked drop of the ST-segment (fig. 6.3 to); generally, this stage lasts few days, maximum two weeks, if it persists more than suspected a complication (aneurysm of the ventricular wall); logically, while more rapid returns the unevenness of ST to the isoelectric line, more pro will be the outcome, although this also will be determined by the presence or not of disturbances of heart rate during this acute phase (extrasystoles, locks, etc.)
2. Sub-acute stage, is recognized by the return of the ST-segment to the line isoelectric, with persistence of a strongly-inverted T wave (fig. 6.3 b); the length of this study is variable, can be extended up to six months.
3. Chronic Stadium, is identified when only persists the Q wave pathological, caused by necrosis, and T-wave is not strongly inverted but flattened or is only slightly negative (fig. 6.3 c).

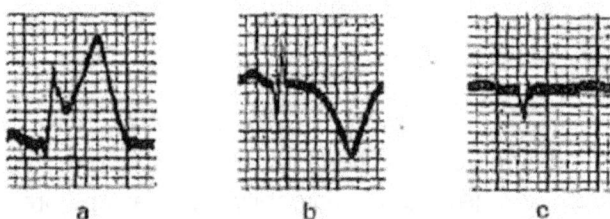

a   b   c

Fig 6.3 evolutionary stages of infarction. Topographic diagnosis or location the topographic diagnosis or location is to determine the area of the heart where they settle the alterations produced by coronary insufficiency, as well as its extension; This often is approximate, every time that the position of the heart can do to vary the relationship of the heart walls with electrodes of different derivations. In general, you can admit that alterations is produced mainly in the anterior face of the heart, in the back or to the side wall of the left ventricle.

The front face of the heart is explored by the precordial V4 VI; the side of the left ventricle by VS, V6, DI, aVL and I diversions to back face, DII, DIII and aVF (fig.6.4) leads.

1. Accordingly, topographical heart disease ischemic and heart attacks can be classified as follows: Anteroseptal, take the front face of the heart in its pretabical portion, the signs appear between leads V1 and V4 (fig. 6.5).

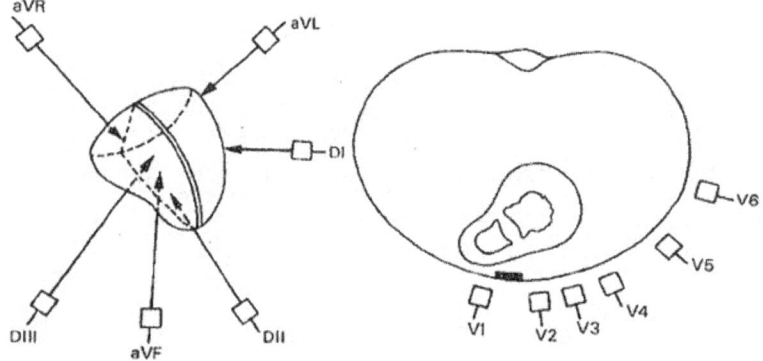

Fig 6.4 heart surface studied by different derivations.

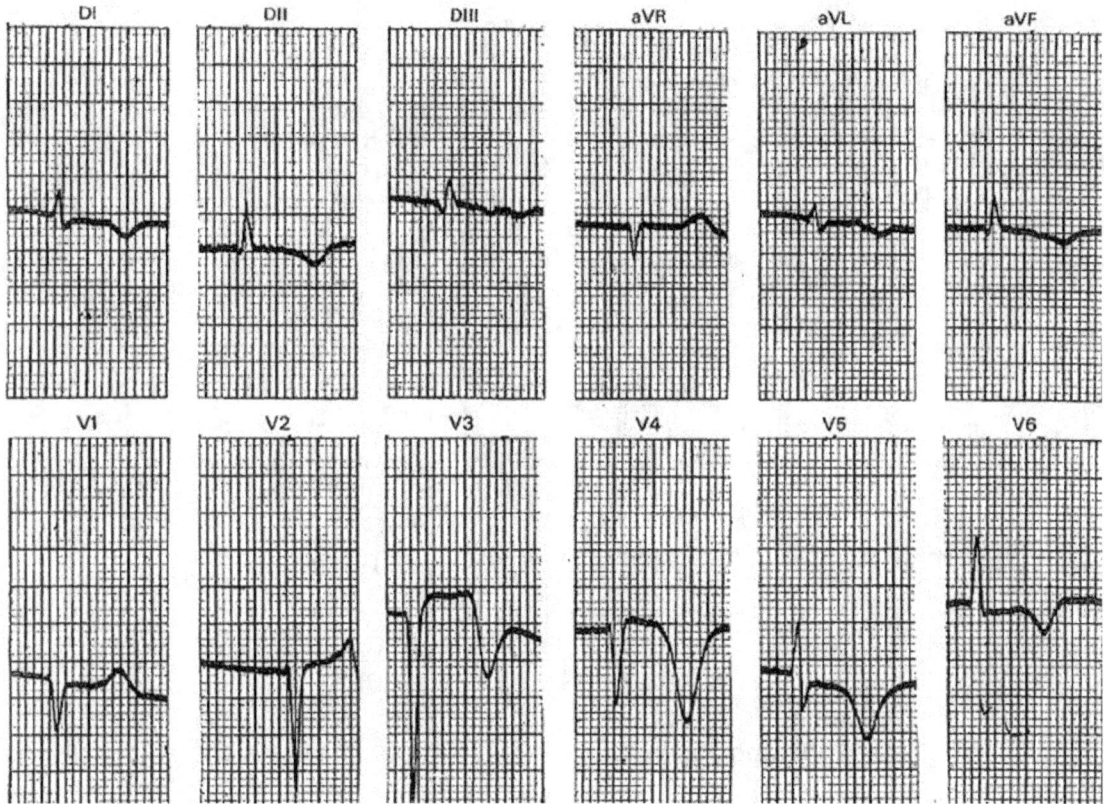

Fig 6.5 Infarct anteroseptal, subacute stage, waves QS in V3 and V4. Ischemia extends also the anterolateral ventricle i border wall. Signs of ischemia (T Waves inverted in DII, DIII and aVF) back.

1. Anterolateral, include the anterolateral side of the left ventricle, the signs are identified in leads V5, V6, DI and aVL.
2. Extensive prior, are a combination of the two described above; symptoms appear between derivations VI and V6, as well as in DI and aVL.
3. Posteroinferior or diaphragmatic, the signs are present in the derivations DI, DIII and aVF (figs: 6.6 and 6.7).
4. Posterolateral, signs can be seen in the DII, DIII, leads to VF yV6.
5. Side altos, identified the signs only in derivations DI and aVL.
6. Sub endocardial, the infarct is opens toward the inner surface of the heart and gives only indirect signs (negative slope of the ST-segment with markedly positive T-wave) in some of the precordial.
7. Intraluminal, pathology (infarction) sits on the inside of the muscle mass and collected strongly inverted T waves and in some of the precordial symmetrical.

Finally, alterations can be diffuse, i.e. range both at the back and in the former or the left side (fig. 6.8).

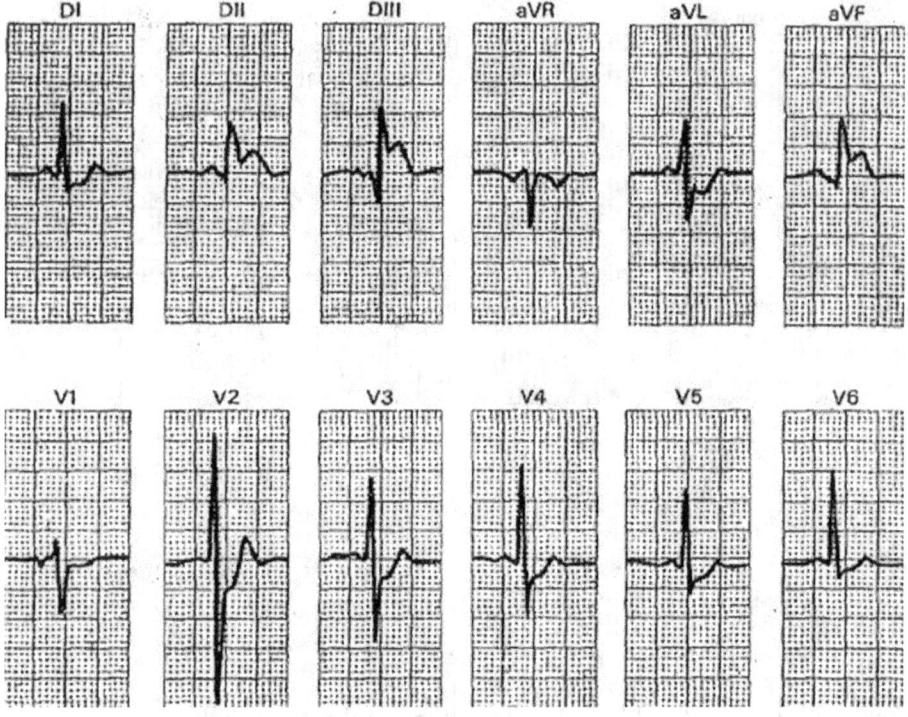

Fig 6.6 Infarction of back or diaphragmatic in acute Stadium, great positive slope of the DII, DIII and aVF ST segment.

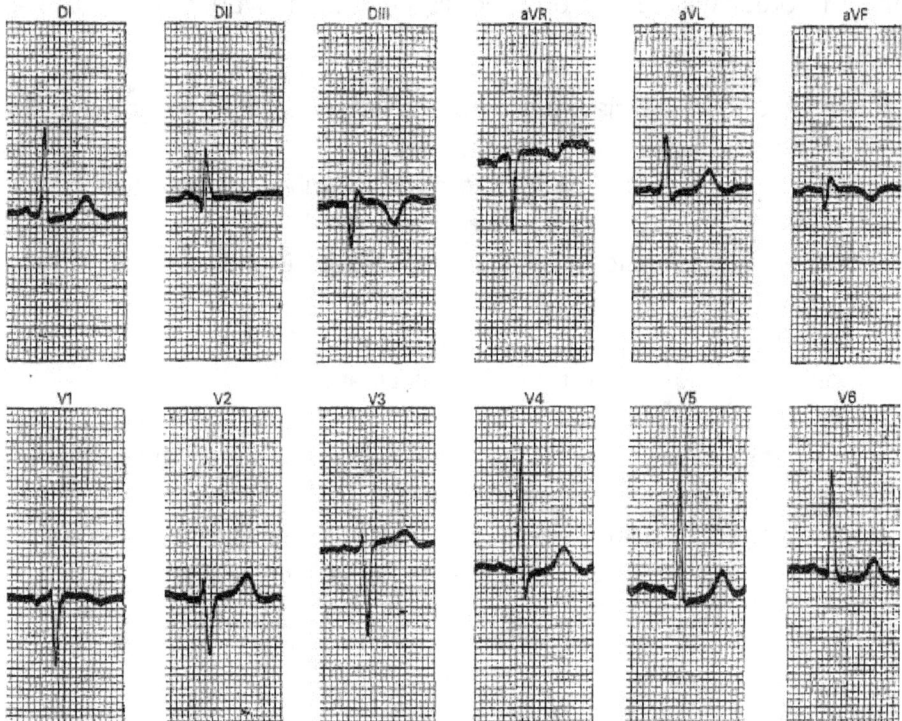

Fig. 6.7 Infarction of myocardial backside in subacute or not recent stage. Pathological Q waves at DII, DIII and aVF with inverted T waves. There is no gap in the ST segment.

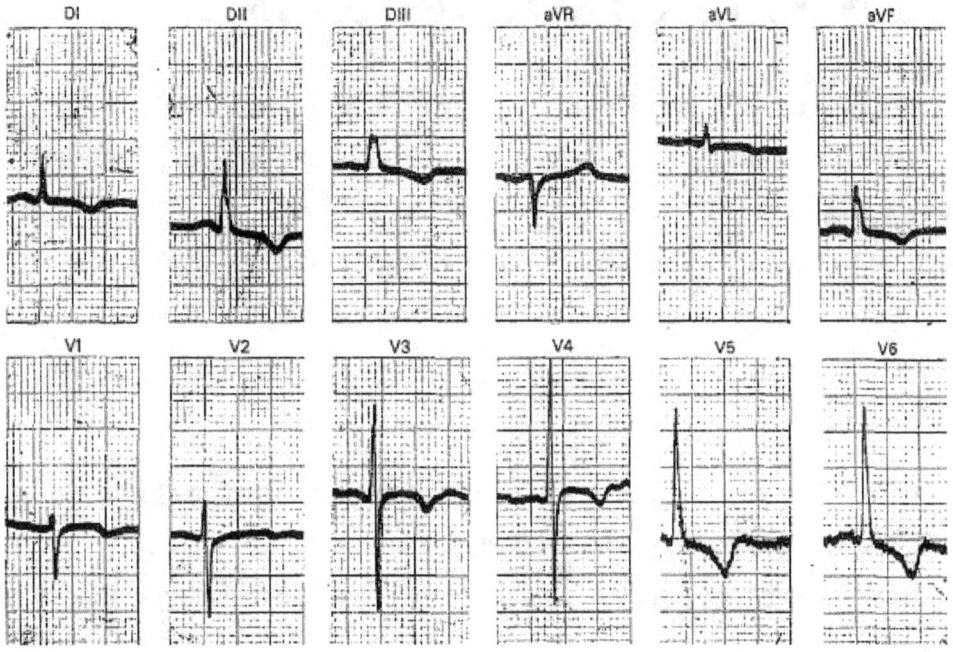

Fig. 6.8 Signs of diffuse myocardial ischemia. T-wave inversion in leads V1-V6, DI and aVL. There are also inverted T waves in the back side DII, DIII and aVF.

7 CHILDREN'S ELECTROCARDIOGRAM

Children's ECGs in the child show some differences in comparison with adult ECG's. This is due to the physiological predominance of the right ventricle, particularly in sucking children and children below the age of 2 years.

The physiological predominance of the right ventricle affects primarily the electric axis and precordial series patterns.

ORIENTATION OF THE ELECTRIC AXIS

In the majority of children, the electric axis tends to occupy vertical positions. In general and depending on a child's age, the electric axis in children may be summarized as follows:

Agreement with age, can be summarized as the axis power in the child is placed in the following way:

• Children 0 to 1 month old, between +30 and +150° (fig. 7.1 a.).

• Children 1 month to 2 years old, between +30 and +120° (fig. 7.1 b).

• Children older than 2 years old, between 0 and +90° (fig. 7.1 c).

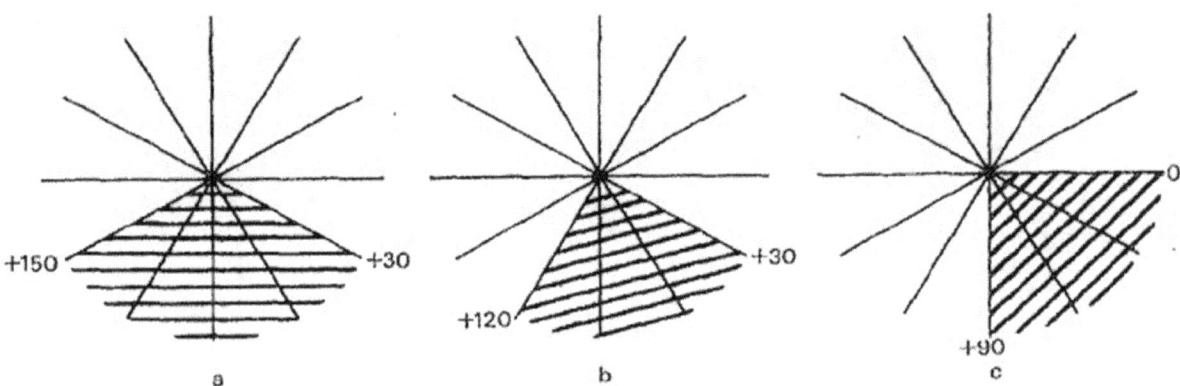

Fig. 7.1 Normal electric axis for children of several ages.

Occasionally, at any age, axes can be seen that are located much to the left, due to the blocking of bundle branch left anterior fascicle.

It is good is remember that exes deviated to the right axis exhibit QRS patterns with a predominance of negative DI and positive DIII. Now, when in that condition, the DII derivation pattern is zero, the axis is to far to the right, +150°. This can be normal only in a child born less than One month ago; but if the pattern of DII is predominantly negative, this means that the axis is more than apart than +150°, which is pathological, even at this age.

When the child is older than one month old, the axis may be more deviated to the right, but not much. That is to say, predominantly negative patters in DI and positive in DIII. In order to determine whether or not the axis is at 120° or more, one needs to use the aVR derivation:
• If it is on an axis deviated to the right the aVR derivation shows an isodiphasic QRS pattern. The axis is at 120°.
• If this pattern is predominantly positive, it indicates that the axe is more apart from 120°, which is pathological in children older than 1 month of age.

Normal patterns in the precordial series

In children, physiologically of right ventricular predominance leaves its footprint in the patterns of the precordial series:

• The R wave in VI is greater than the S wave in the age of 2 years.
• This preponderance is greater with younger and younger children.

In general terms, one can say that in the newly born less, than a month old, the R/S normal progression of the adult is inverted, in such a way that there is a predominant R wave in Right derivations VI, V2 and V4r* and a predominantly S wave in the left precordial derivations V5 and V6 (fig. 7.2 a.).

In children between the ages of one month and two years of age, partial inversion usually exists, with dominant R waves in the right precordial derivations and also on the left precordial derivations (fig 7.2b).

For children older than 2 years old, the regular adult progression pattern is gradually established, with a gradual increase in the magnitude of R-wave, while the electrode moves from right to left in the precordial zone (fig. 7.2 c)

Occasionally, there may be some children slightly older than 2 years, in whom the R wave predominates over the S wave on the VI derivation.

V4r. A derivation taken from the fifth rib space at the level of the median clavicular line, which must be performed on children due to the possibility of a dextrocardia.

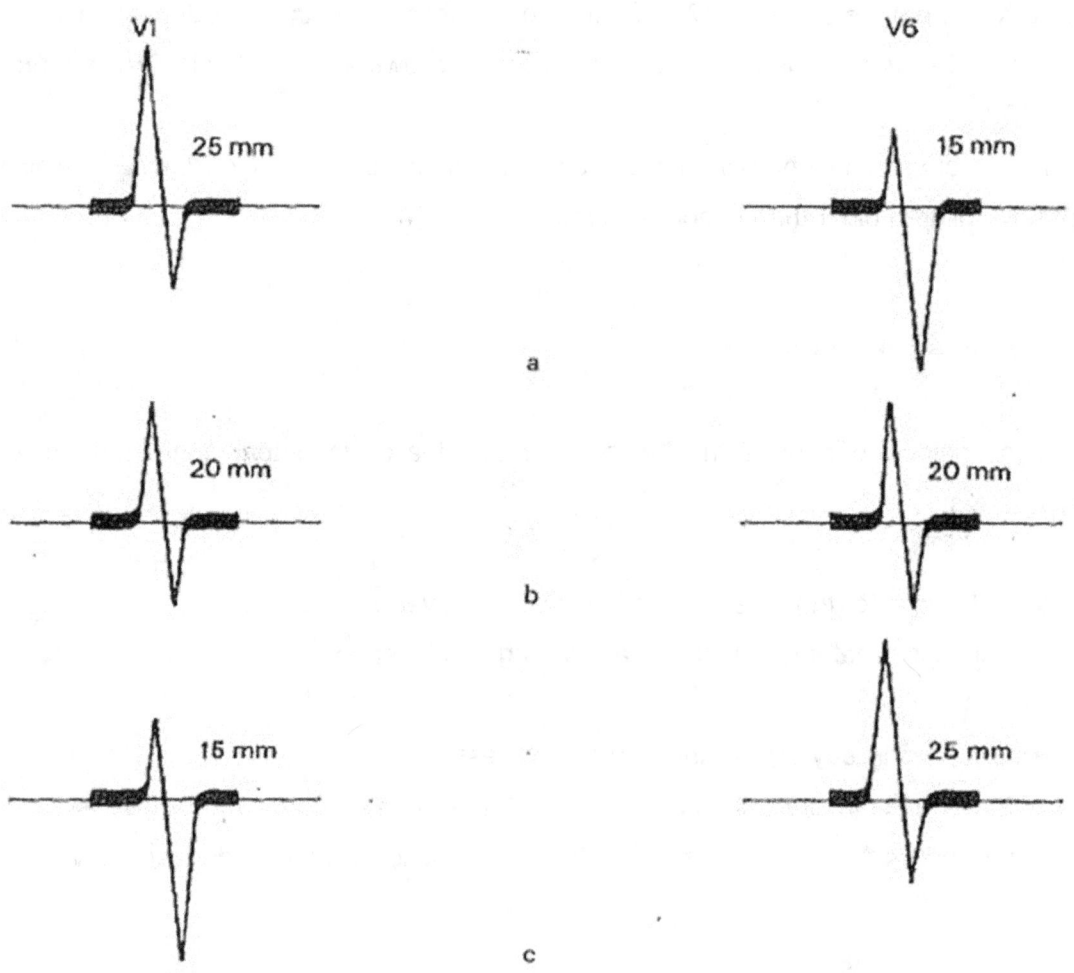

Fig. 7.2 normal patterns in precordial derivations VI and V6 in children of different ages.

The P wave
There are no significant differences in relation to the ECG P wave for an adult.

The PR Interval

Normal values of the PR interval in children vary with age and heart rate; normal measurement of this interval is shortened as heart rate increases, but in general terms it can be said that a PR interval greater than 0.1 s in children is overextended. In general, the PR interval does not exceed 0.12s in children younger than one year old.

Extended, shortened alterations or fixed duration of the PR interval in children are the same as described for adults.

The QRS Complex

In terms of orientation of the QRS complex electric axis. It has already been said in the child, due the right ventricle physiological prevalence, the axis may be something more to the right than usual; and normal values of these deviations were analyzed according to age.

As regards to the QRS complex voltage, it was also explained which voltages are normal in the precordial series with different ages, however, is appropriate to highlight that, since children have thorax walls that are thinner than same in adults, children generally show higher voltages than adults in the precordial series; so for example. The Sokolow index, which is considered normal up to 35 mm in adults, in children older than 2 years it is up to 45 mm; in children the less than 2 years old, because a physiological right ventricular predominance exists, once again validates the number of 35 mm.

As soon as the duration or width of the QRS complex, a child generally is below 0.08 s and tends to decrease with younger children.

As in the case of adults, minimum figures are not of interest. The QRS width is stretched in the bunch Branch blocks in the Wolff-Parkinson-White syndrome and, occasionally, in ventricular hypertrophy.

The ST Segment

In children, as well as in adults, a positive or negative displacement of the ST segment is of much interest. In vagotonic children, a positive difference in levels may occur, which may be accompanied by strongly positive T waves; in acute pericardities, flattened T waves are added; in severe necrotizing myocarditis the type or anomalies occurring in coronary arteries, inverted T waves additionally occur.

The ST segment negative difference in levels may be observed in cases of digitalis intoxication (vat ST) or in pathologies that produce myocardic hypoxia.

The T wave

The T waves show one more difference between children's and adult ECGs. In children, T waves are normally negative on the right precordial derivations V4r, V1, V2 and V3 (also, occasionally, V4) in almost children and these conditions may remain with children until they have reached their second decade of age (the juvenile pattern); however, during the first 24 to 28 hours of life, the T wave is generally positive on the right precordial derivations and may be inverted on the left precordial derivations,

There is a group of anomalies in children that may produce an inversion in the T wave on those derivations on which the T wave must obligatorily be positive (V5, V6, DII and DIII), such as:

- Endocardic fibroelastosis.
- Acute myocarditis in suckling.
- Glucogenesis.
- Anomalous left coronary origination.

The T waves may be high voltage and symmetric in hyperpotassemia, vagotonic individuals, left ventricle diastolic overloads, in addition to the recovery phase of rheumatic myocarditis.

Electric alterations in the most common cardiopathies

Non-cyanotic with an increased pulmonary flow.

C.I.A.
It produces an ECG that, in more than 90% of cases, shows a pattern of an incomplete right bunch Branch block, with polyphasism on right precordia's; the axis appears to be somewhat deviated on the first quadrant, which may point to an first degree AV block.

Large C.I.V.
Some signs of left ventricle diastolic load. Alternatively, some signs of combined ventricular hypertrophy may appear.

Large P.C.A.

It indicates left ventricle diastolic overload and, more commonly, it indicates signs of combined hypertrophy.

Severe Aortic Stenosis

There are some signs of severe left ventricular overload (sinking of the ST segment, with flattened or inverted T waves on left derivations); some signs of right overload may appear due to pulmonary hypertension.

Severe aortic compression

Usually, there are some combined ventricular hypertrophy, with left or right predominance.

Cyanotics with pulmonary normal or diminished flow

It is designed to would complement radiology, helping make the differential diagnosis even more precise.

The cardiopathy of this group. Causes without cardiomegaly

Tetralogy of Fallot:

The trace shows P waves of pulmonary morphology and signs of ventricular hypertrophy. The axis rarely goes beyond the +150°. Voltages on the V and V4.r may be highly altered, but, as something very characteristic, the V2 derivation shows a deep S and, above all, the T wave is strongly positive in this derivation.

Common core with diminished F.P.

The electrocardiogram will show more or less manifest right ventricular hypertrophy, although it may not be helpful to establish the differential diagnostic between theses two entities, it is essential to resort to other specialized investigations.

Atresia and stenosis with decreased tricuspid F.P.

An electrocardiogram is highly valuable since it is the only group cardiopathy that runs with an electrode that shows signs of left ventricular hypertrophy, and a left axial deviation. The P waves are wide and high and show a notch on its cusp. However, the P wave alterations may not be very visible in subjects until 3 or 4 years of age.

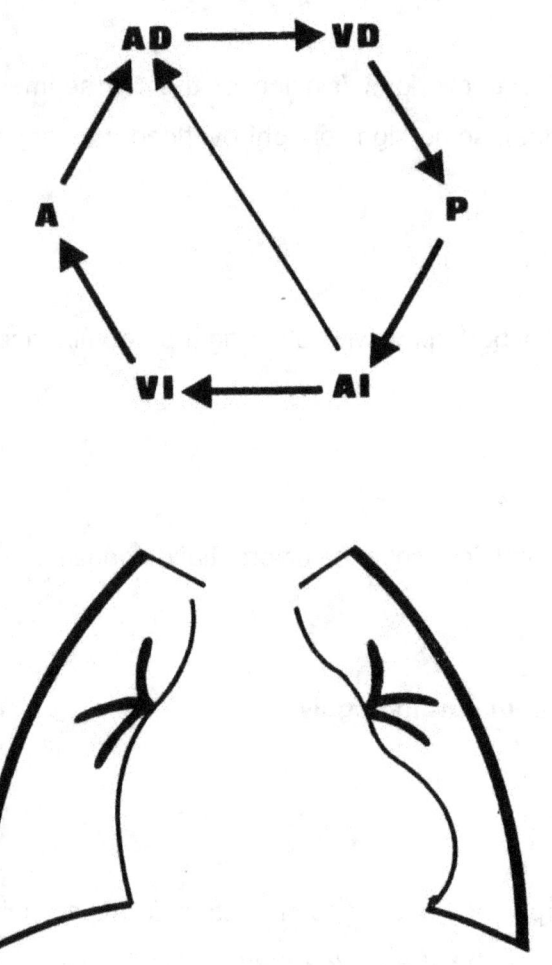

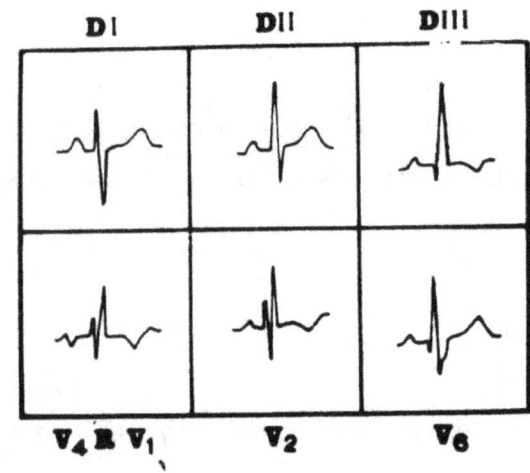

Fig. 7.3 Big C.I.A.

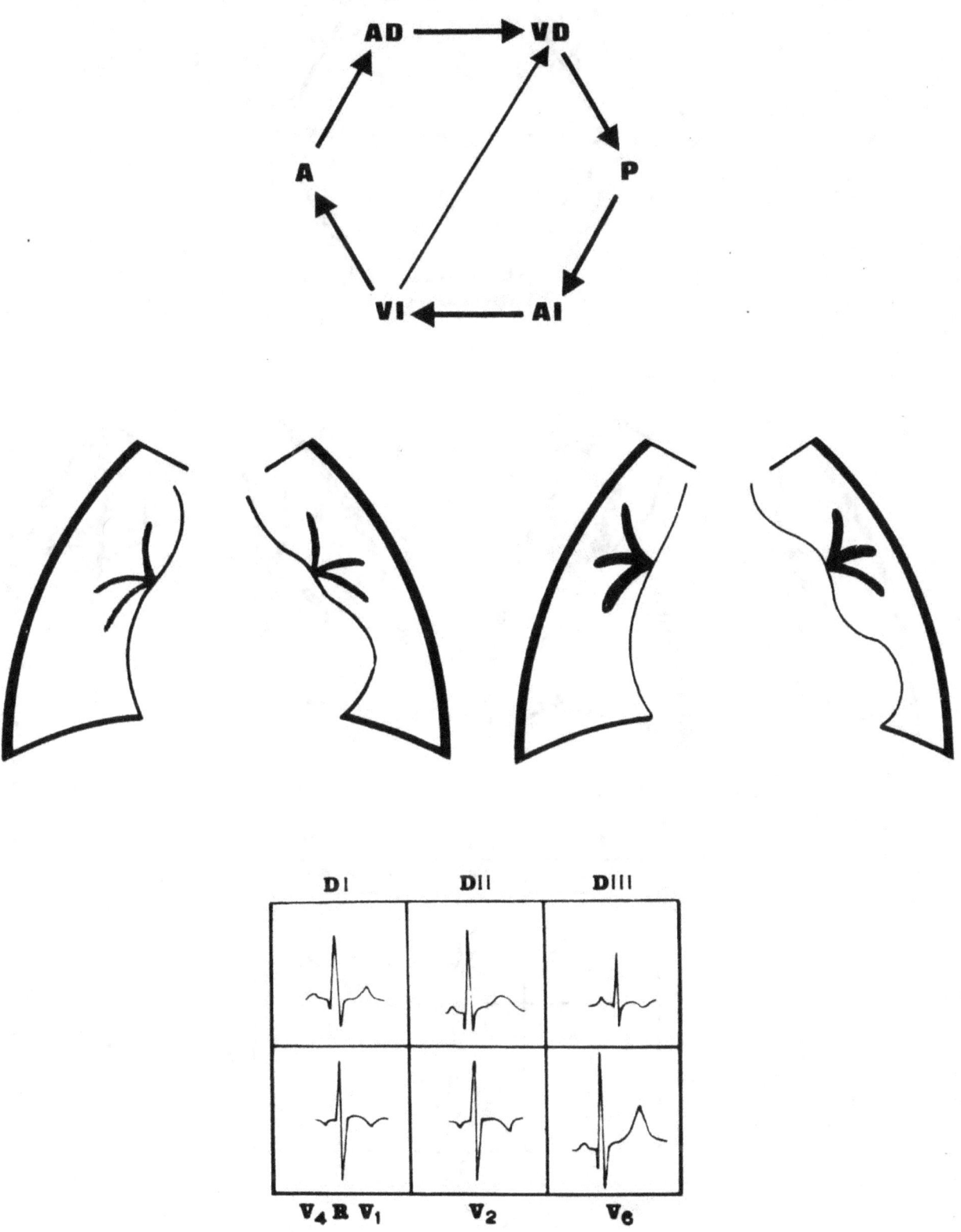

Fig. 7.4 Big C.I.V.

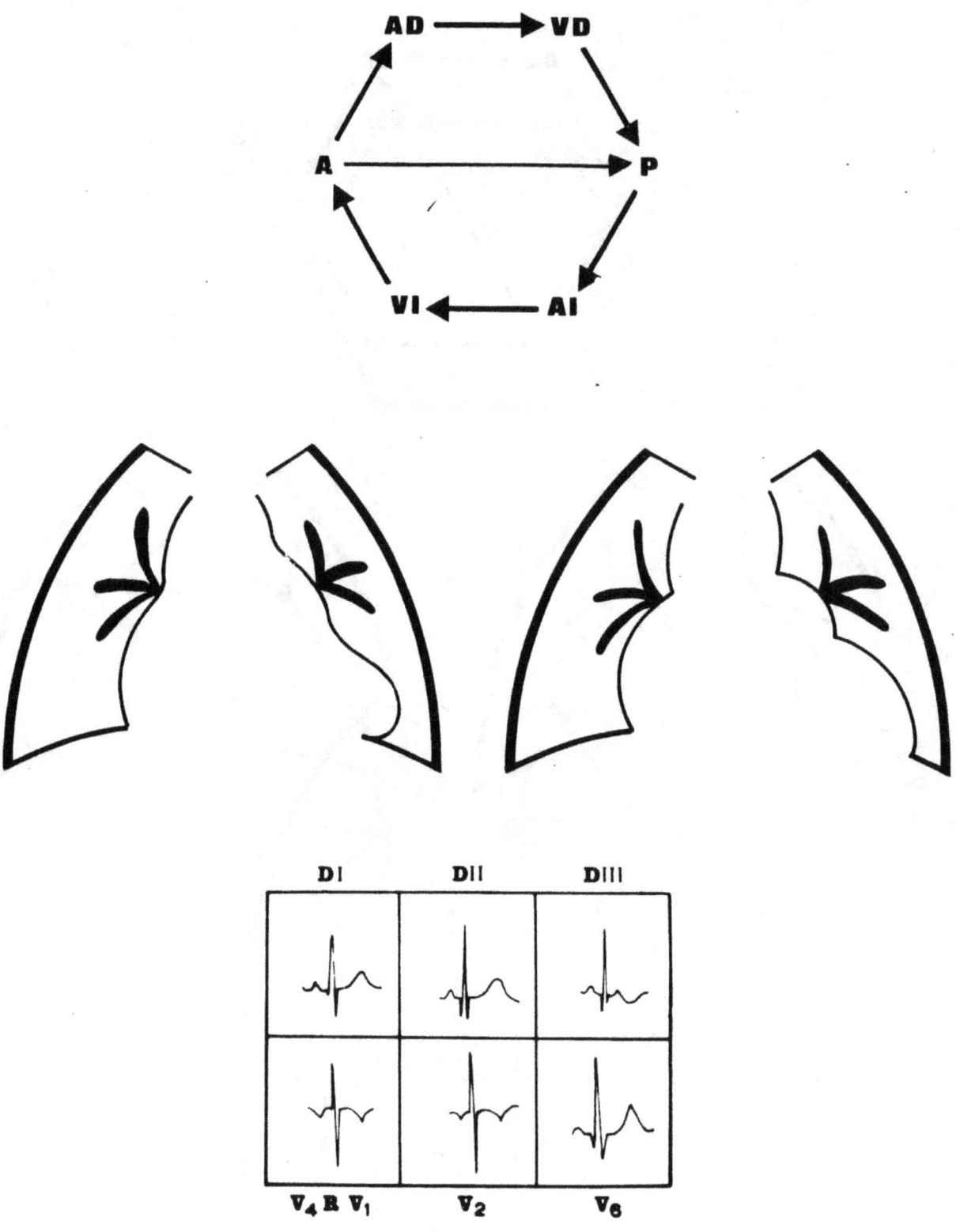

Fig. 7.5 Big P.C.A

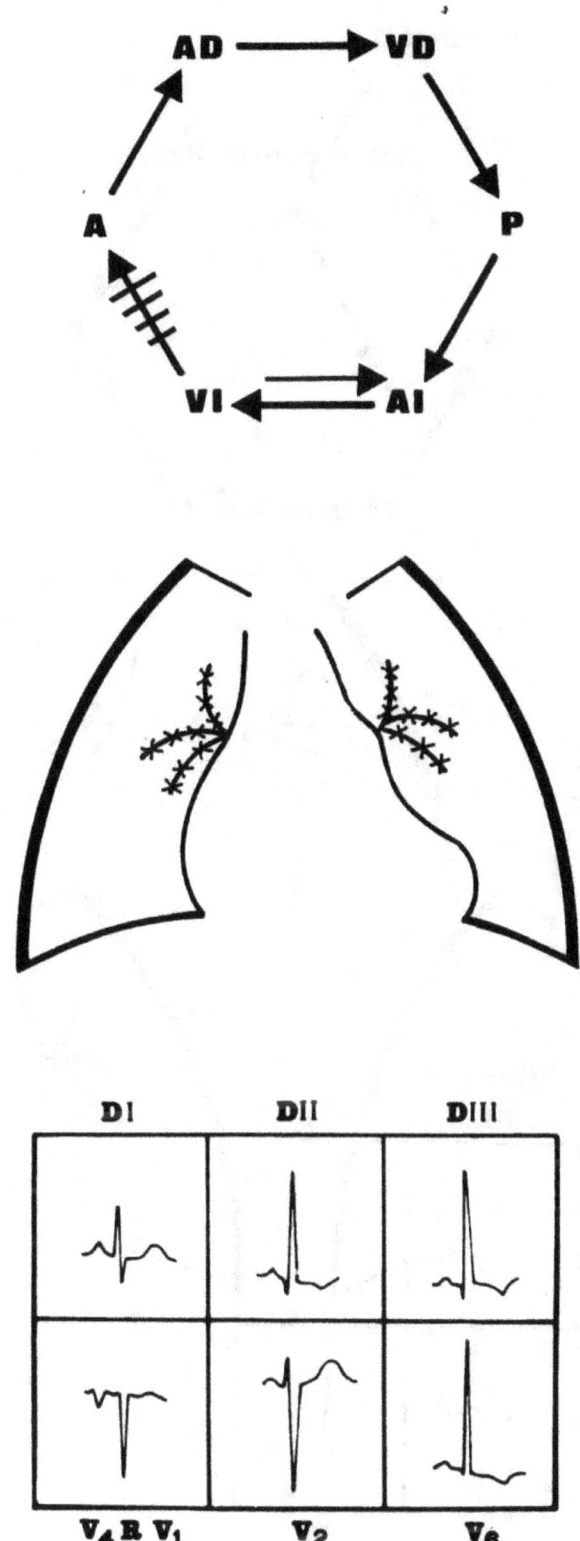

Fig. 7.6 Severe aortic stenosis.

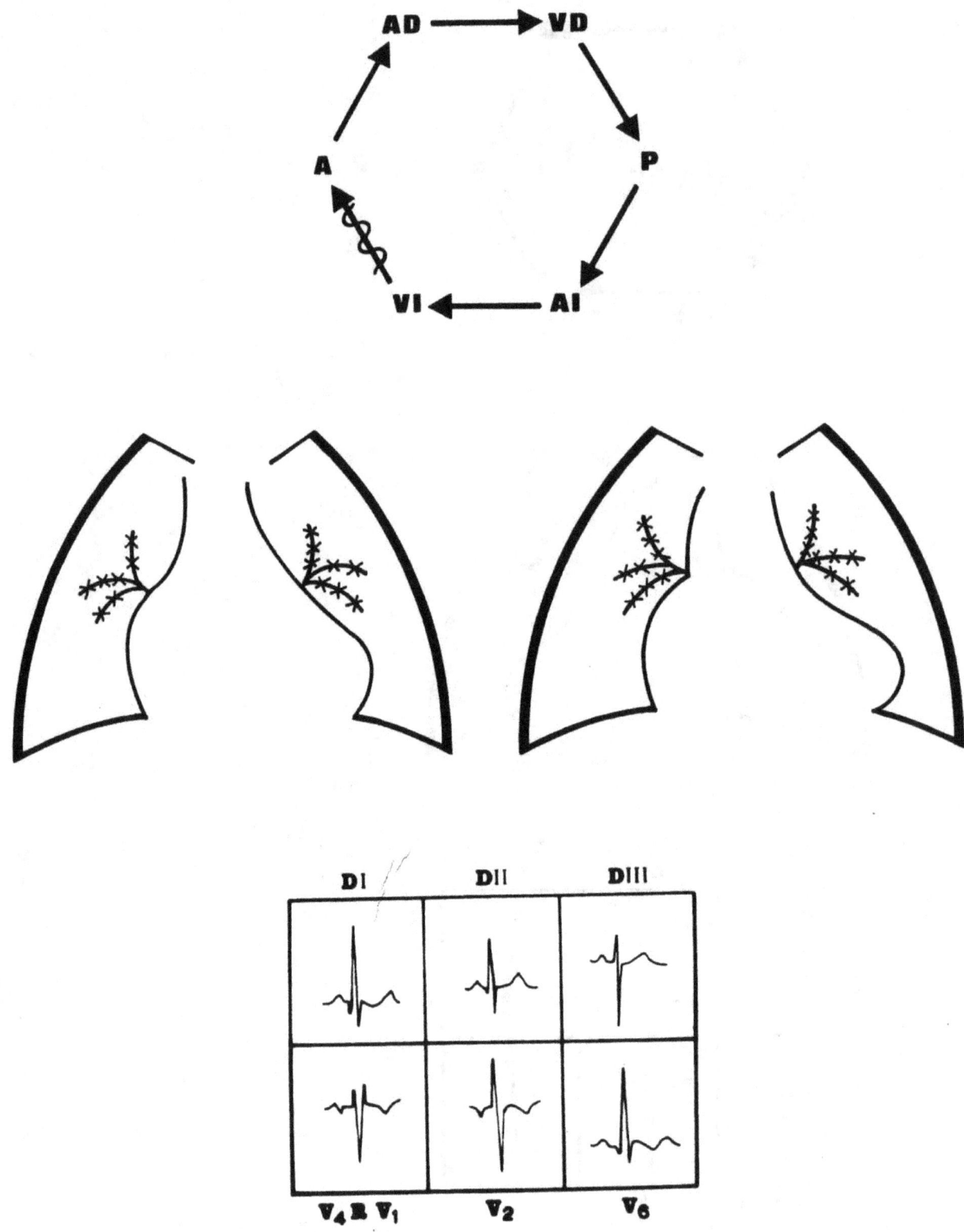

Fig. 7.7 Severe aortic coarctation.

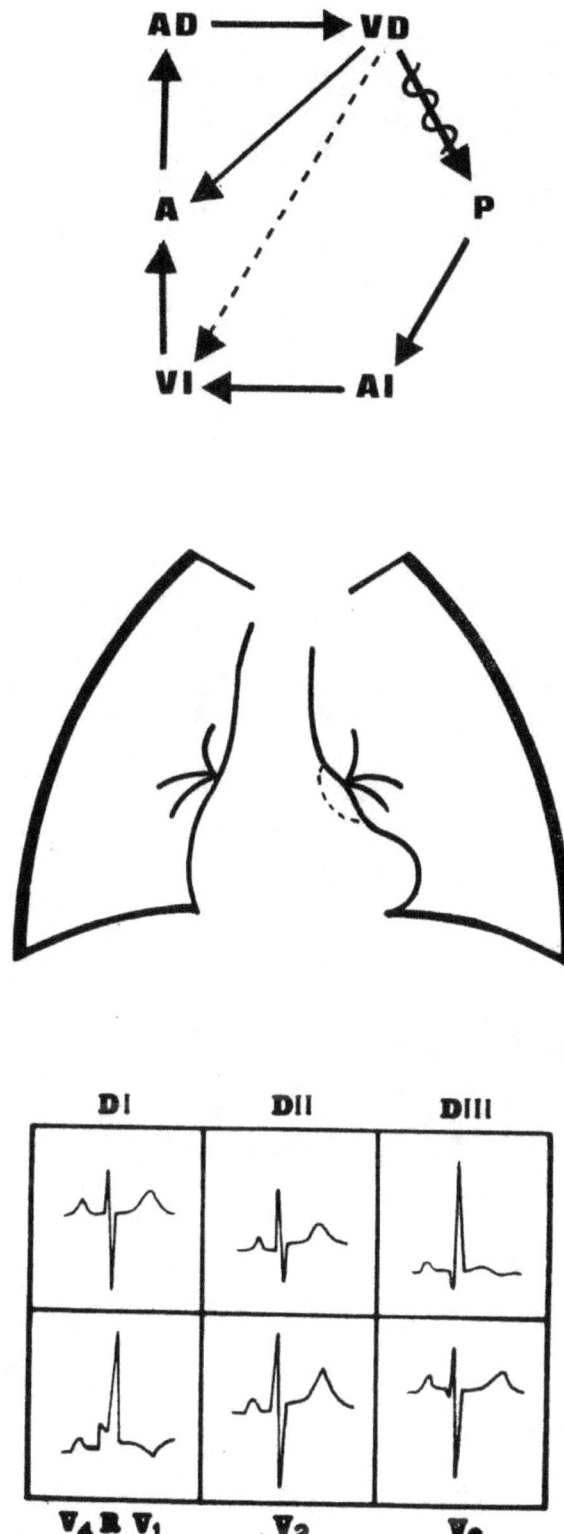

Fig. 7.8 Tetralogy of Fallot

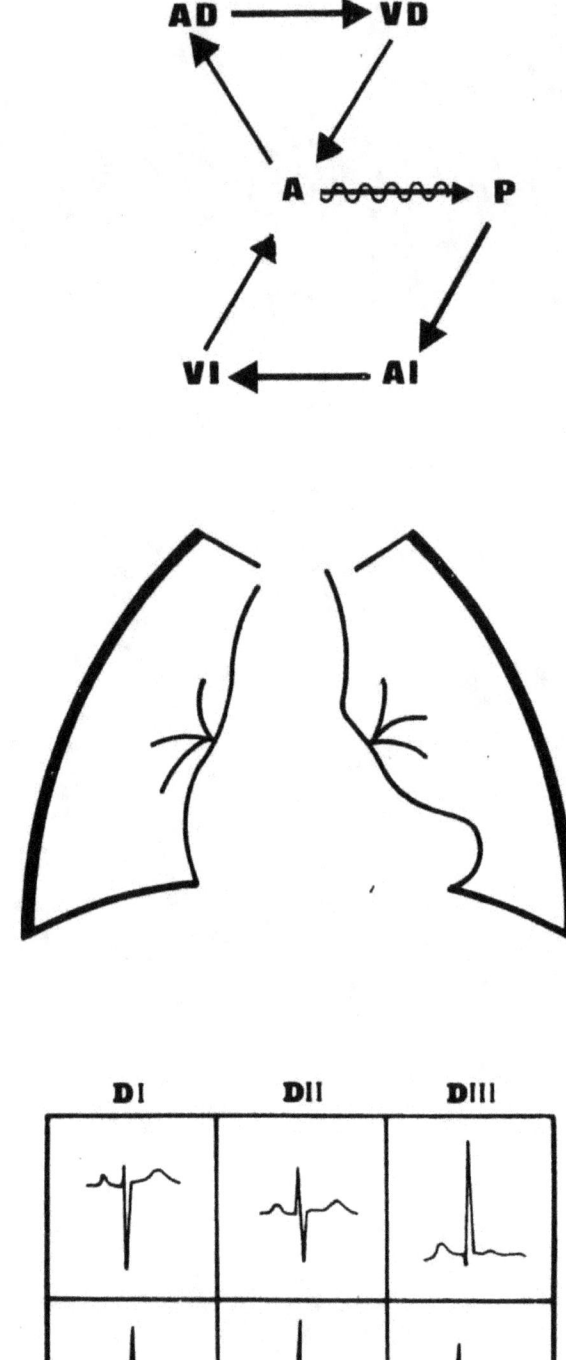

Fig. 7.9 Common stock with F.P decreased

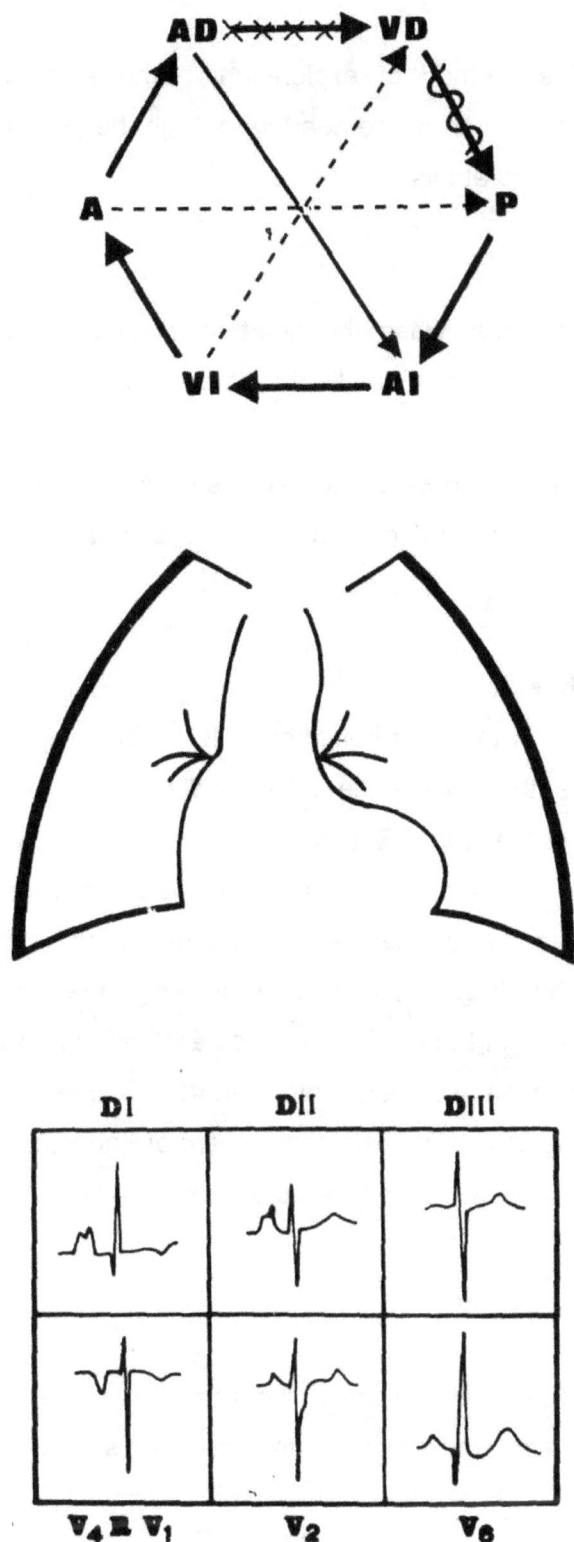

Fig. 7.10 Tricuspid stenosis and atresia with F. P. diminished

ELECTROCARDIOGRAMS IN DEXTROCARDIAS

The electrocardiogram is extremely valuable method of exploration in the study of the dextrocardia, not only in the recognition of the position of the heart in the right hemithorax, but also, in the diagnostic of the relative position of the atrials and the ventricles because, as is well known, there are two major dextrocardia types:

- The so-called true one with *situs inversus,* when the heart is located in the right hemithorax and the heart chambers (right auricles and ventricles are located on the left, and viceversa).
- False dextrocardia, also called dextroversion, in which the heart, is located in the right hemithorax, but the heart chambers are not interchanged, i.e., the right auricles and ventricle rights are to the right.

Diagnostic of the heart position on the right side.

The presence of the heart abnormally located in the right hemithorax. Is easily settled, when observes to the negative prevalence all waves (the P wave, the QRS complex and the T wave). Usually the QRS complex exhibits a pattern of the type QR: there are, however, one needs to be cautious, because this morphology un the DI derivation may also be due to an error when making the electrocardiogram, by having exchanged the cables corresponding to the arms. To resolve this matter, one needs to resort to the study of the patterns shown in the precordial series: if the patterns show a normal progression in the precordial series and the right ventricle patterns V1 and V2 are verified, in addition to those of the left ventricle in V5, V6, one is dealing with a mistake in placing the cables; now in the case of a dextrocardia there are no variations in the pattern of the precordial series, although the voltage decreases as the electrode moves to the left and away from the heart this is minor.

Diagnostic of relative auricle position

As regards the relative auricle position, the presence of a frankly negative P wave on DI and positive on DIII indicates that the auricles are inverted, because, in this case, the stimulus (the P vector) is oriented from left t right (fig. 7.11).

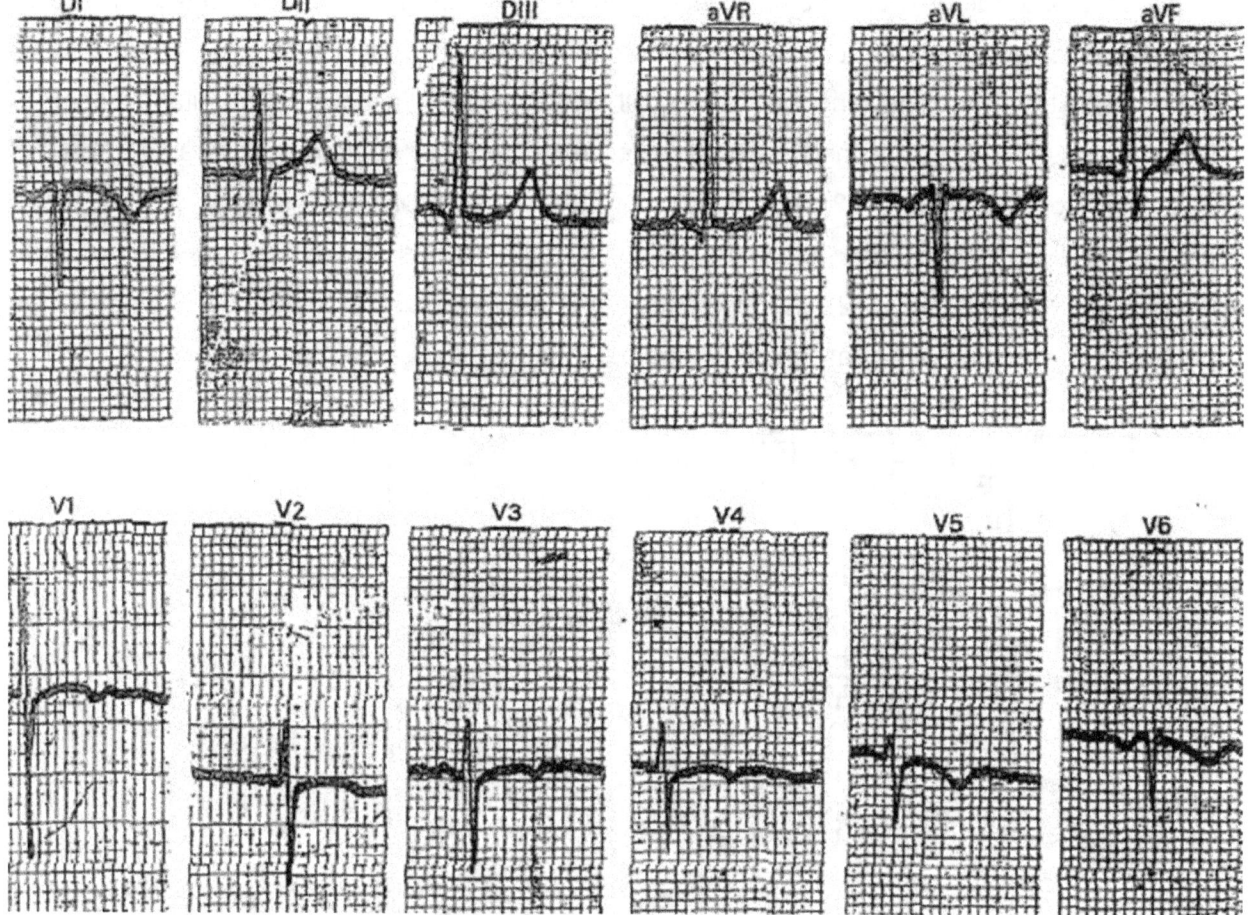

Fig. 7.11 Dextrocardia with situs inversus. The predominantly negative DI derivation , ARS and T; in the precordial series, the V1, V2 and V3 derivations show predominantly negative patterns (right ventricle), that persist all the way to V6, although the voltage is less).

When the auricles are in a normal position, the P-wave is not strongly inverted on DI, but it tends to be flattened, since in this case the auricular or vector P activation goes from right to left, but, since the heart is located in the right hemithorax, and the tip of the heart is on the right, the result is that the P vector is perpendicular to the DI derivation (fig. 7.12).

Diagnostic of relative ventricle position

As regards relative ventricle position, it is easy to determine it based on a study of the precordial series, provided that the right ventricle patterns are known to be predominantly negative or double R, while those of the left ventricle begin with a small negative wave but are predominantly positive.

In the case of a true dextrocardia or a *situs inversus,* the pattern picked up from the V1 and V2 derivations is that of the right ventricle (predominantly negative or in double T) and the same patter persists in the remaining derivations, all the way to V6, although the voltage becomes less and less (fig. 7.11). In the case of a false dextrocardia or cardiac extroversion, the QRS that shows on the V1 and V2 derivations is of the left ventricular type (begins with Q and is predominantly positive) and holds on the entire precordial series all the way to V6, with diminishing voltages (fig. 7.12). In these cases, it is also very useful to conduct a study of the patterns shown on a precordial series, carried out to the right.

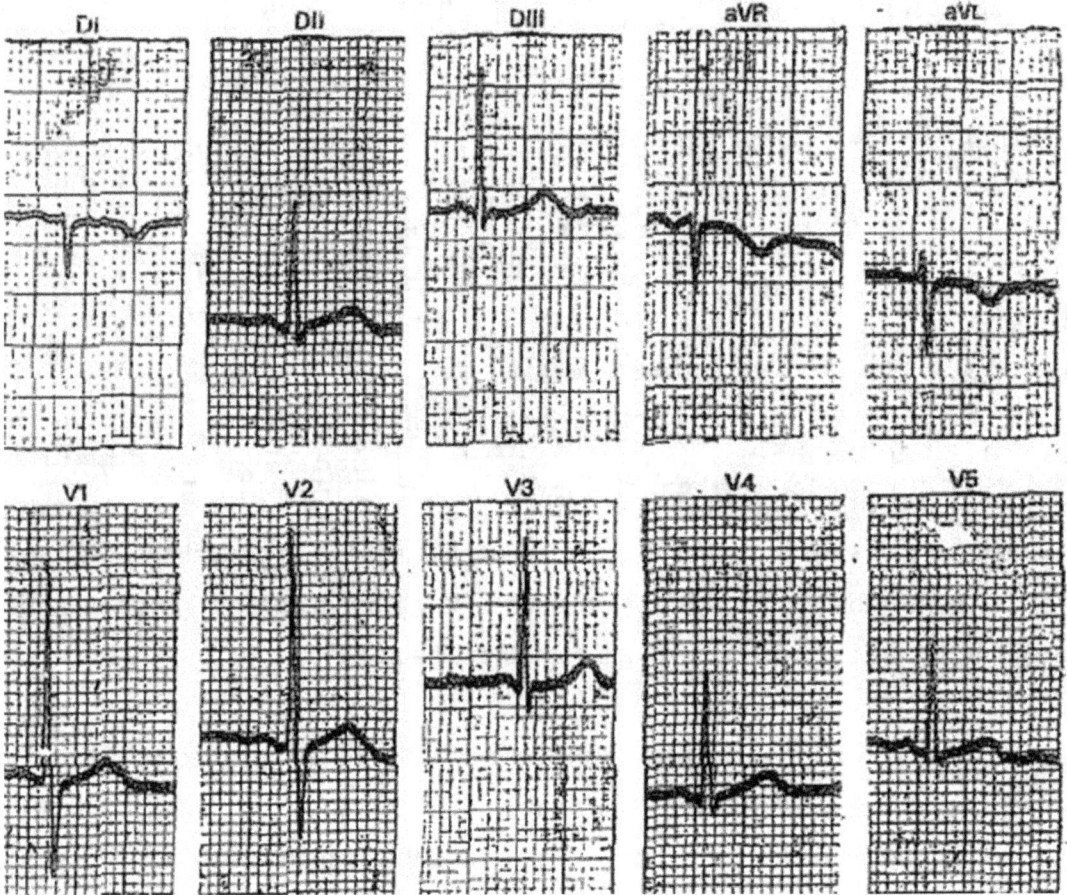

Fig. 7.12. False dextrocardia or cardiac dextroversion. The DI derivation with a flattened P wave, QRS and T predominantly negative; the QRS patter of V1, V2 and V3 is that of the left ventricle and persists all the way to V6, although with lesser voltage, that is, the ventricle is located on the left.

References

1. Electrophysiology: The Basics: A Companion Guide for the Cardiology Fellow during the EP – October 26, 2009 by Jonathan S. Steinberg MD
2. Textbook of Medical Physiology: With STUDENT CONSULT Online Access, 11e – September 1, 2005 by Arthur C. Guyton, John E. Hall
3. Rapid Interpretation of EKG's, Sixth Edition – October 15, 2000 by Dale Dubin
4. 12-Lead ECG: The Art Of Interpretation – November 13, 2013 by Tomas B. Garcia
5. Epidemiology of atrial fibrillation: European perspective. Clinical epidemiology 6: 213–20. Zoni-Berisso, M; Lercari, F; Carazza, T; Domenicucci, S (2014).
6. Cardiac Arrhythmias: Their Mechanisms, Diagnosis, and Management (3 ed.). Mandel, William J., ed. (1995).
7. The value of electrocardiogram for the cardiological diagnosis in the XXI Century. VOLUME VII - NUMBER 12014; 7: 13-40 WRITTEN BY Andrés Ricardo Pérez-Riera M.D. Ph.D1.; Frank G. Yanowitz, MD2.
8. ECG in Emergency Medicine and Acute Care. Elsevier Mosby 2005. Chan TC, Brady WJ, Harrigan RA, Ornato JP, Rosen P.
9. The ECG Made Easy. 7th edition. London: Churchill Livingstone 2008. Hampton JR.
10. Pediatric Cardiology for Practitioners. 5th edition. St Louis: Mosby 2007. Park MK.
11. Electrocardiography in Clinical Practice. 6th Edition. Saunders Elsevier 2008. Surawicz B, Knilans TK. Chou's.
12. Coexistence of right bundle branch block high-grade and right ventricular pre-excitation paraseptal later does the simultaneous ECG diagnosis is feasible? Milagros María Caro, Alexander Caneva, Hugo A. Garro, Rafael S. Acunzo, Paul A. Chiale; Cardiac Arrhythmia Center of the City of Buenos Aires. Cardiology Division. Acute General Hospital J.M. Ramos Mejia and - Institute Sacre Coeur. Buenos Aires, Argentina.Type A Wolff-ParkinsonWhite syndrome obscured by left bundle branch block associated with a vascular malformation of the coronary sinus. Br Heart J 1988; 60:352- 354. Robinson K, Davies MJ, Krikler DM.
13. Electrocardiographic characteristics of patients with Ebstein's anomaly before and after ablation of an accessory atrioventricular pathway. J Cardiovasc Electrophysiol 2006;17:1332-1336. Iturralde P, Nava S, Sálica G et al.
14. Wolff Parkinson White syndrome in Ebstein's disease. Arch Inst Cardiol Mex 1955; 25: 17-34. Sodi Pallares D, AJ Soberon, Cisneros F, Seafood F, Alvarado A.
15. Ebstein Anomaly: clinical profile in 174 patients. Arch Inst Cardiol Mex 1999; 69: 17-25. Attie F, Casanova JM, Zabal C, et al.
16. Electrocardiographic characteristics of patients with Ebstein's anomaly before and after ablation of an accessory atrioventricular pathway. J Cardiovasc Electrophysiol 2006; 17: 1-5. Iturralde P, Nava S, Salica G et al.
17. Coexistence of right bundle branch block high-grade and right ventricular pre-excitation paraseptal later. Electro RV and Arrhythmias 2010; 2: 63-68 Caro MM, Caneva A, Garro H, R Acunzo, Chiale PA
18. Atrioventricular block - First degree AV block - PR interval, Second degree AV block - Type 1, Third degree AV block, From Wikipedia, the free encyclopedia

19. ECG recording during atrioventricular block (in Spanish). Walgreens drugstores
20. Coronary ischemia, From Wikipedia, the free encyclopedia
21. "Sacred Heart Medical Center: Spokane, Washington : Coronary Ischemia:". Shmc.org. Retrieved 2008-12-28.
22. "Cardiac Ischemia Symptoms." LiveStrong. Demand Media, 9 Mar. 2010. Web. 6 Nov. 2010. Potochny, Evy.
23. "Coronary Artery Disease." Adult Health Advisor (July 2009): 1. Consumer Health Complete. Web. 4 Nov. 2010. RelayHealth.
24. "Ischemia." Ischemic Heart Disease. Ischemic Heart Disease, n.d. Web. 6 Nov. 2010.
25. "Diagnosis of Coronary Heart Disease." Hopkins Heart (Jan. 2008): 18-25. Consumer Health Complete. Web. 17 Nov. 2010. Gerstenblith, Gary, and Simeon. Margolis.
26. "Lifestyle Measures to Prevent and Treat Coronary Artery Disease." Hopkins Heart (Jan. 2008): 25-36. Consumer Health Complete. Web. 29 Nov. 2010. Gerstenblith, Gary, and Simeon Margolis.
27. Myocardial infarction, From Wikipedia, the free encyclopedia
28. "ESC Guidelines for the management of acute myocardial infarction in patients presenting with ST-segment elevation.".European heart journal 33 (20): 2569–619.
29. "Sex differences in symptom presentation in acute myocardial infarction: a systematic review and meta-analysis.". Heart & lung: the journal of critical care40 (6): 477–91.
30. "Prevalence, incidence, predictive factors and prognosis of silent myocardial infarction: a review of the literature". Arch Cardiovasc Dis 104(3): 178–88.
31. "Heart Attack or Sudden Cardiac Arrest: How Are They Different?". http://www.heart.org/. Jul 30, 2014. Retrieved 24 February 2015
32. "Ischemic heart disease in women: A focus on risk factors.". Trends in Cardiovascular Medicine25 (2): 140–151.
33. Global atlas on cardiovascular disease prevention and control (PDF) (1st ed. ed.). Geneva: World Health Organization in collaboration with the World Heart Federation and the World Stroke Organization. pp. 3–18.
34. "Acute myocardial infarction". Lancet 372 (9638): 570–84. White HD, Chew DP; Chew (August 2008).
35. "Women's early warning symptoms of acute myocardial infarction".Circulation 108 (21): 2619–23. McSweeney JC, Cody M, O'Sullivan P, Elberson K, Moser DK, Garvin BJ (2003).
36. Acute Coronary Syndrome American Heart Association. Retrieved November 25, 2006
37. Electrocardiography, From Wikipedia, the free encyclopedia
38. "Einthoven's String Galvanometer: The First Electrocardiograph". Texas Heart Institute journal / from the Texas Heart Institute of St. Luke's Episcopal Hospital, Texas Children's Hospital 35 (2): 174–8. Rivera-Ruiz M, Cajavilca C, Varon J (29 September 1927).
39. "Un nouveau galvanometre". Arch Neerl Sc Ex Nat 6: 625. Interwoven W (1901).
40. Atlas of cardiovascular monitoring. New York: Churchill Livingstone. Mark, Jonathan B. (1998).
41. RESTING 12-LEAD ECG ELECTRODE PLACEMENT AND ASSOCIATED PROBLEMS. DrTanzi
42. "Electrocardiogram explanation image". Retrieved 28 February 2014.
43. Cyanotic heart defect, From Wikipedia, the free encyclopedia

44. Step-Up to Medicine (Step-Up Series). Hagerstwon, MD: Lippincott Williams & Wilkins. Page Elizabeth D Agabegi; Agabegi, Steven S. (2008).

45. Revised content Congenital Heart Disease by Dr. Vicente Montagud Balaguer, Medical Specialist in Cardiology Hospital Consortium General Universitario de Valencia. Bachelor of Medicine and Surgery at the University of Valencia. Last Review: February 2015

46. Epidemiology of congenital heart disease. F. Moreno 2005 [cited 2010].

47. History and physical examination in pediatric cardiology. Madrid2005 Santos de Soto J. [cited 2010].

48. Role of pediatric cardiologists in the management of neonates with congenital heart disease. Arch Pediatr2001 Oct; 8(10):1121-4. Marcon F, Bosser G, Lucron H, Lethor JP.

49. Patent ductus arteriosus and aorto-pulmonary window. Madrid2005 [cited 2010]. Medrano.C., Zavanella C.Tetralogy of Fallot: from fetus to adult. Heart 2006 92: 1353-1359

50. Congenital heart disease. In: Bonow RO, Man DL, Zipes DP, Libby P, eds. Braunwald's Heart Disease: A Textbook of Cardiovascular Medicine Webb GD, Smallhorn JF, Therrien J, Redington AN

51. Dextrocardia, From Wikipedia, the free encyclopedia

52. On the differentiation of two forms of congenital dextrocardia. Bulletin of the International Association of Medical Museums (5): 134–138. M. E. Abbott and J. C. Meakins (1915).

53. Kartagener Syndrome, Renee A Laux MS

54. Clinical Vignette: Dextrocardia with Situs Inversus: Through the Looking Glass with an ECG. Proceedings of UCLA Healthcare (Department of Medicine, UCLA) 15, Bindra, S. MD Tabibiazar, R. MD Mazar, M MD and Dave, R MD (2011).

55. Cecil Textbook of Medicine, 2-Volume Set, 25e, Goldman-Cecil Medicine May 11, 2015 by Lee Goldman MD and Andrew I. Schafer MD